PRAISE FOR *LIMITLESS*

"Mimi's story shows you should never give up. If things don't go your way, you can adapt and move on."

Nell McAndrew, author and fitness enthusiast

"What a great read! Truly inspiring. This book highlights how ordinary people can achieve extraordinary things by using resilience and determination to turn disappointment into future success. I challenge anyone to read it and not be inspired to go out and challenge themselves to overcome their own limits."

Aly Dixon, Olympian and 50 km World Champion

"In Limitless, *Mimi shows that sometimes the greatest adventures in life come from finding the courage to step away from our dreams and into the unknown. Her story is refreshingly honest and powerful – an inspiration for anyone who's just starting out, or looking to start all over again."*

Anna McNuff, author and adventurer

PRAISE FOR *BEYOND IMPOSSIBLE*

"This book will inspire you to take on new challenges and achieve things you never believed you could... While you might not be up to world-record attempts or super-ultra-length runs, Mimi will inspire you to be brave enough to take that next step on your running journey."

Leanne Davies, Founder of Run Mummy Run

"A heart-warming story full of unimaginable feats."

Lisa Jackson, author of *Your Pace or Mine?*

LIMITLESS

An Hachette UK Company
www.hachette.co.uk

Summersdale Publishers Ltd
Part of Octopus Publishing Group Limited
Carmelite House
50 Victoria Embankment
LONDON
EC4Y 0DZ
UK

www.summersdale.com

Printed and bound in China

ISBN: 978-1-78783-634-1

Substantial discounts on bulk quantities of Summersdale books are available to corporations, professional associations and other organizations. For details contact general enquiries: telephone: +44 (0) 1243 771107 or email: enquiries@summersdale.com.

Some of the names of those involved in Mimi's adventures have been altered for this book.

LIMITLESS

AN ULTRARUNNER'S STORY OF PAIN, PERSEVERANCE AND THE PURSUIT OF SUCCESS

MIMI ANDERSON

WITH LUCY WATERLOW

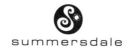

summersdale

CONTENTS

PROLOGUE

June 2019

I woke up on race day full of dread. My stomach was churning with butterflies and my heart was pounding. Eating breakfast was definitely out of the question as I felt so nervous. All I could manage was a coffee – most unlike me ahead of a physical challenge.

I had already laid out the kit I would wear the night before, and had packed everything else I would need into my bag (double-checking it was all there more than once throughout the evening). All I needed to do was get dressed and go, but I kept checking everything again which was delaying my departure. My husband, Tim, kept looking at his watch wondering why it was taking me so long to leave.

"Shouldn't you have left by now?" he asked.

He has always been fully supportive of my sporting endeavours – no matter how ambitious. And this challenge was arguably one of my most outlandish. A sprint triathlon. I have made a name for myself as a Guinness World

Record breaking ultrarunner. "Sprint" is not usually in my vocabulary. I had so many doubts swirling around my mind.

I can't go, I thought. *I'm not ready, and I don't know if I ever will be. I don't think I can do this.*

I'm not usually one to be so defeatist before I've even tried something. In the past, I have thrived on proving to myself and others that I can do things that seem impossible. But at that moment, I didn't feel like the formidable sportswoman I once was. I had been through a lot in the previous two years that had knocked me down both physically and mentally. I now didn't know if I had the strength or ability to become a triathlete.

If you want something you have never had, then you have to try something you have never done, I thought to try to psych myself up. This was the mantra that had led me to sign up for the Cranbrook Triathlon in Kent, held in June 2019, in the first place. It entailed a 300 m (328 yd) pool swim, 21 km (13 mile) bike ride and 5 km (3.1 mile) run. Out of the three disciplines, there wasn't one I felt fully confident about. I was a nervous swimmer, an apprentice cyclist, and a runner returning from injury. Then there were the transitions. The thought of them was especially daunting. Some say triathlon is actually a four-discipline sport, not three, because of everything you need to do and remember in transitions between the swim, cycle and run. Races can be won or lost based on how quickly you can go through them without incurring any penalties. There was a lot to think about, much more so than doing an ultramarathon race, which is often just about getting from A to B. In ultras where I had a crew, I never had to think about anything other than running. They planned and provided everything for me, from helping me change my kit when needed, to plying me with snacks and drinks. In the triathlon, I would be on my own.

I kept telling myself it didn't matter how messy and amateurish my transitions were, or how slow my bike ride and run were. All that mattered was finishing, never mind the time it took. And then I had another thought – I could be worrying myself over the transitions needlessly, as I might not even make it that far to do them. In order to cycle and run, first I would have to swim. And this was my greatest fear of all. The thought of swimming in a competitive environment was absolutely terrifying. I was worried about being able to control my breathing while doing front crawl – a technique I had only recently learnt. I was petrified of the other swimmers who would be splashing and bumping into me as they swam with all their might to go as fast as they could. But most of all, I was worried about simply being in the water. This wasn't just usual pre-race nerves, it was a debilitating anxiety. It stemmed from a childhood incident where I witnessed my younger sister, Jacqui, almost drown in an icy river. She survived unscathed but the experience scarred me for life. Being near or in water immediately makes me recall the horror and helplessness I felt that day.

They say you have to face your fears to truly defeat them, and that's why I had entered the triathlon race to try to do just that. I was now 56 years old. I had avoided it for long enough. It was time to dive in and finally overcome my phobia. So, I picked up my kit bag and told Tim I was off, even though I wanted to stay at home. He gave me a hug and wished me luck, then came to help me put my stuff into the car.

Come on Mimi, you can do this, I told myself as I headed out the door. When I put my mind to a long-distance running goal, I was determined to see it through. I now had to apply that same determination to triathlon. I racked up my bike on the car as Tim put my bags on the front seat. All I needed to do now was get myself in and go, but as I went to open the car door, my resolve wobbled again.

"I can't go," I told Tim.

"Really?" he said with surprise. "You're not going to try?"

He knew I had been preparing for this for weeks, and I wasn't usually a quitter. I thought about it some more. I really didn't want to do it. But at the same time, I knew how disappointed I would be with myself if I didn't. If I stayed at home, I would be kicking myself for the rest of the day, and only end up entering another triathlon. Not only that, my friends from Weald Triathlon Club, that I had joined the year before, were expecting to see me there. Others who followed me online were also waiting to hear how I got on, as I had been sharing my triathlon journey on social media.

How could I tell everyone that I didn't do it because I was too scared? I had even chosen a triathlon with the easier option of a swim in a leisure centre pool over a scarier open water one, but to me it was still just as intimidating. I felt so nervous even thinking about being in the water again, I thought I was going to be sick right there on our driveway. I was on the verge of bursting into tears. How had it come to this? I had once won ultramarathons in the desert and the Arctic, and set world records for running across Britain and Ireland. Now I was ready to back out of a race before even making it to the start line. Petrified, fearful, unsure of myself and what my body was capable of. Could I overcome my fears and become a triathlete?

PART ONE:

RUNNING AMERICA FOR A WORLD RECORD

CHAPTER ONE

THE AMERICAN DREAM

If you had told me in 2016 that becoming a triathlete would be a huge target of mine, I would have thought you were bonkers. I had my long-standing fear of water and was happy to keep avoiding it; I barely rode a bike; and running 5 km (3.1 miles) wasn't challenging for me then. At that time, I was fully ensconced in the ultrarunning world and preparing to take on my biggest challenge yet – attempting to set a new Guinness World Record running across America in the fastest time for a woman. I would start at City Hall in L.A. and finish on the steps of City Hall in New York, running 2,850 miles (4,587 km) in between. I had been working towards this goal for a long time but to say it had always been a dream of mine would be untrue.

I only started running in my thirties and began by barely being able to run a mile on the treadmill. I wouldn't have been able to run across a small park, let alone the third largest continent in the world. Back then I was a stay-at-home mother of three who had only taken up running because I wanted to have slimmer and more toned legs. I never expected running to become such a big part of my life and identity. It was when friends I had made at the gym encouraged me to step off the treadmill and run with them outside that I discovered my passion for running. When running through a forest or along a scenic path surrounded by countryside, I had never felt more free. It made me feel alive and it gave me freedom and space away from being a wife and mum. It also helped me banish an eating disorder that could have killed me in my twenties. Running taught me that food is fuel, not something to fear or avoid. If I wanted to run well, I had to eat well. It also changed my attitude towards my body image. I started caring less about how my body looked and more about what it could do. And what it could do continued to amaze me.

I never thought I would be able to run far but in 2000 I completed my first half marathon, the Hastings Half Marathon. I then ran my first ultramarathon in 2001 – the 54 mile (87 km) Thames Meander. It was a training run for my main goal at that time – the Marathon des Sables. This is a 155-mile (250-km) self-sufficiency race over six days in the Sahara Desert. I thought it would be a great adventure with my newly made running friends, even though I had no experience of running such a long distance in extreme heat. It nearly broke me, but I absolutely loved it. It was there that my love of ultrarunning and pushing myself out of my comfort zone was born. I didn't look back after that, I kept finding myself new challenges.

The seed was sown in my mind to run across America in 2011. I had achieved two Guinness World Records by then. The first was becoming the fastest female to run the length of Great Britain (John o'Groats to Land's End, or JOGLE), running 840 miles (1,352 km) in 12 days, 15 hours and 46 minutes in 2008. Then in 2010, I ran 403.81 miles (649.87 km) on a treadmill in seven days, a Guinness World Record for the greatest distance run on a treadmill in one week by a woman at the time. In both of these challenges, I had loved the whole process of making and then executing a plan to achieve my goal. Of course, there were times when I was in extreme pain, and low moments where I questioned whether I could do it, but the hardship made the feeling of accomplishment when I did succeed even sweeter. The pride, joy and relief at pushing myself beyond my perceived limits to gain a new world record felt like nothing else. I was keen to see what else I could achieve on a global scale.

I had been following the progress of a fellow ultrarunner and friend called James Adams who had been taking part in the LA–NY (Los Angeles to New York) Footrace. As I followed the highs and lows of his journey via his blog, I thought it sounded fantastic. It ignited a flame inside me, and I knew that one day I would tackle my own journey across America. The goal had been set. It would be the ultimate test of my running ability. But having decided that was my goal, it was another six years before I was ready to do it. These sorts of challenges need a huge amount of planning, preparation and fundraising, not to mention the training, and there were setbacks getting my body into the best condition to face such an arduous run.

The time to beat

The record I was aiming to beat had been unbroken for decades. It was set by South African Mavis Hutchison, who ran coast to coast in 69 days and 2 hours in 1979. My aim was to try to run it in 50 days. (I worked out this would mean running about 57 miles / 92 km per day. That's nearly 399 miles / 642 km per week for just over seven weeks.) But I told the world via social media that I was aiming to do it in 53 days, as I thought this would take the pressure off, and give me room for manoeuvre in case of any unexpected hold-ups. This might sound like crazy mileage, but it wasn't an unrealistic goal for me given my previous endurance feats. I had gained a third Guinness World Record in 2012 with the fastest crossing of Ireland on foot, where I ran a total of 345 miles (555 km) in three days, 15 hours, 36 minutes.

On top of the world record challenges, I had also completed many of the world's toughest ultras as doubles. This involved taking part in the organized race with the other competitors. Then after having a very short break at the finish, I would turn around and do the entire course again in reverse, just me and my support crew. In 2009, I was the first female to do the double at Comrades, South Africa, a total of 112 miles (180 km); in 2011, I completed double Badwater in California's Death Valley, a total of 292 miles (470 km); in 2013 I became the first person to run the double at the Grand Union Canal Race between Birmingham and London (having previously broken the female course record in 2010), a distance of 290 miles (467 km); and in 2015, I was the first female to complete the double Spartathlon, Greece, a total of 306 miles (492 km). The furthest I had ever run in a challenge was in 2014, when I ran 1,223 miles (1968 km) in 32 days along the Freedom Trail in South Africa from Pietermaritzburg to Cape Town. I knew I would have to draw on all my previous experiences to get me through the run across America, and I was confident in my ability to do it. Completing endurance events in extreme conditions had become my speciality.

People often ask me, why America? Why not another country or a different world record? It is largely because crossing America is so iconic in endurance sports. It is known as one of the toughest challenges an ultrarunner or long-distance cyclist can take on – and many try and fail. I also loved the idea of running coast to coast, something I had enjoyed when I ran from the top to the bottom of the UK, and across Ireland. You simply can't beat touring a country on foot. It is a unique opportunity to really see places you might otherwise never visit and meet people whose paths you would never cross in everyday life.

Another part of the appeal is that the country is so vast, with changing terrain and extremes of weather as you go through the various states. I could expect to face blistering heat, strong winds and heavy rain along my way. There is also a risk of snow, but this is less likely if you attempt the crossing in spring or autumn. I had run ultras in mountain ranges, deserts, jungles and the Arctic before, so I felt prepared for whatever altitudes and temperatures lay ahead. In a way, I felt as though everything I had done before had been building up to running across America. On a lighter note, I would often joke to my friends that I have always wanted to go to New York but Tim wouldn't take me, so I would just have to run there instead!

The route

The most intricate aspect of the preparation lay in plotting the fastest possible route across an entire continent that contains mountain ranges, canyons, gigantic lakes and protected National Parks. My plan had always been to start at City Hall in L.A. and finish on the steps of City Hall in New York. There are a few ultrarunning enthusiasts in America who like to call this the "easy" route (actually, they have another name for it but that's too rude to write here!) as it is shorter than running from San Francisco to New York. It also involves less elevation (although the route I chose would still rise to over 10,000 feet / 3,048 m above sea level).

My reason for choosing this route was quite simple. Mavis had run from L.A. to New York to set the original record so, to me, it seemed only natural that I should start and finish in the same places. This was confirmed in my mind when, shortly after announcing my intentions, I received an unexpected message from Mavis's daughter wishing me good luck, and telling me that both she and her mother would be following my progress. It would be an honour to attempt to follow in her footsteps.

Knowing I wanted to run from L.A. to New York was one thing, but actually working out how I would do it was quite another. To begin with, I simply used an online map to plot a walking route, putting the respective City Halls in as my first and final destinations, which would be approximately 2,800 miles (4,500 km). This gave me a rough outline of the path I could take, but it would need a lot of tweaking.

My original plan had been to start the record attempt in September 2016. I was incredibly lucky to be able to go to the USA in the May of that year to drive the route, along with Tim and a two-man film crew from Scrumptious Productions who were going to document my world record attempt. Carol Cooke, Scrumptious Productions founder and creative director, had discussed the possibility of making a documentary about me after she heard me giving a talk at an event in Edinburgh. I briefly shared my story, from taking up running in my thirties to becoming an accomplished ultrarunner, and finished by speaking about my plans to run across America. Carol came to speak to me afterwards and, over a glass of Prosecco, she said she thought filming my record attempt would be an amazing opportunity to document what goes into a challenge of this magnitude. Like me, Carol is passionate about inspiring more women to exercise and we agreed this would be a wonderful way to do it.

"It is such an amazing story," she said of my journey to become an ultrarunner. "And to be able to film you in action as you take on your next challenge would be so exciting and show people what really goes into running a world record. I would love to witness it for myself and capture it to show others."

I was extremely flattered that Carol was so interested. I agreed with her – I would love to show people that anything is possible. I was just a mother of three who took up running because I wanted slimmer legs and now I was going to run across America. I wanted to show that anyone can do great things if they put in the time and effort and believe in themselves. However, I warned Carol that being on the road with me for more than 50 days would be gruelling. There would be early starts and long days, and I wouldn't want any of the filming to interrupt my or the crew's routine. Carol assured me that they wouldn't get in the way. She hoped we would quickly forget they were there with their cameras, as she wanted everyone to act naturally. They would travel in their own RV which she would organize and fund herself.

There didn't seem to be any reason to refuse so I welcomed her aboard. Carol and another member of her team called Graham decided to come on the May recce so they could start getting a feel for what shots they could do and to get to know me better before the run. It was important I felt at ease talking to them and Carol wanted to film the preparation that went into a world record attempt.

On the road trip, we covered approximately 350 miles (563 km) each day. Seeing the journey I was preparing to take from the comfort of a car brought home just what an epic challenge I was taking on. I would be running through 12 states: California, Nevada, Arizona, New Mexico, Colorado, Kansas, Missouri, Illinois, Indiana, Ohio, Pennsylvania and New York, and within four time zones (starting in the Pacific, then crossing into the Mountain, Central and Eastern zones) losing an hour of sleep each time. The drive-through recce was essential for fine-tuning the route, as we discovered that some sections, particularly in the Western States, would be inaccessible to the support vehicles I would have travelling with me, or went through private land including Native American reservations.

Under Guinness World Record rules, it is forbidden to take a route through private land unless you have prior permission. At one stage we drove through farmland in Colorado where we had to find the owner to get permission to pass. We stopped outside a house to be met by three guys, a father and his sons drinking tea out of jam jars. Carol in her broad Glaswegian accent tried to explain what we were doing, he just looked blankly at her (she does talk very fast!) so Tim took over. One of the men then very kindly rang up the owner and got permission for us to run through the farm in September (although in the end we decided not to use this route). Just as we were about to leave the father took great delight in showing us the marijuana plants he was growing, as it's legal to do so in that state as long as you are a resident, over 21 years old, and only cultivate up to six plants. We were not sure if he was just proudly showing off his efforts, or trying to sell us some! To change the subject, we admired a large bison he had in one of his fields which he told us was called Pisser. When we asked why, he replied: "Because he's always so pissed off!" That did make us laugh as we continued on our way.

Another rule of Guinness is that you cannot run along interstate highways as it is far too dangerous. So, throughout the trip, we were constantly having to seek alternative suitable roads, while trying to keep the mileage as low as possible. Eventually we had a route we were happy with which was a total distance of about 2,850 miles (4,587 km).

The road trip involved sitting in the car for hours on end, but I did make time to fit in a run each day to stretch my legs. This gave me a wonderful taste of the experience I had to come. The scenery everywhere we went was stunning. We drove through arid desert land, along winding mountain roads, through lush forests and past rolling green fields that stretched away for miles. The sky above was always huge and I was constantly marvelling at what a massive country the USA is. The highlight of the journey was driving over the George Washington Bridge in New York where I saw the Manhattan skyline for the first time. I felt a wave of emotion come over me as I imagined myself running over the bridge in September, so close to completing my journey on the steps of City Hall. I like to "bottle" these thoughts and emotions in my mind so I can draw on them when I'm going through a bad patch and need a kick up the backside.

After sampling a few cocktails in New York and running around Central Park (something I had always wanted to do) we returned home shattered but excited about the adventure that lay ahead, along with copious amounts of notes, photos and maps covered in lines we had drawn and redrawn.

The crew

The next stage in the preparations was to ensure I would have an amazing crew to support me every step of the way. I would need people I could trust; who understood ultrarunning and who were willing and able to give up weeks of their time to accompany me. A world record attempt is all about teamwork. They would be in charge of keeping me on the right route, laying my kit out each evening for me to wear in the morning, feeding me and keeping me company at certain points during the day as I ran (making sure they always ran beside or behind me, but never ahead, as that would be deemed as pacing, as per Guinness World Record rules). The crew would also be responsible for collecting the evidence for Guinness to ratify a world record, should I achieve one. This would include obtaining signatures from witnesses along the route who had seen me run past, taking numerous videos, and logging all breaks and stops to sleep. There were many rules and regulations I would have to stick to and I needed my crew to be on top of them all. It would have been soul destroying if I achieved a world record only for it to be officially denied due to a technicality.

There have been some high-profile cases in ultrarunning involving people who claimed to have run records, only to be exposed as cheats. I wanted my record attempt to be honest and transparent so providing all the necessary evidence to prove it was essential. My crew would be responsible for this, along with absolutely everything else that needed to be done, allowing me to focus solely on the running. Although it wasn't required by Guinness, I would also wear trackers while I was running to monitor my progress and so that people could follow my journey online.

It didn't take long to assemble my marvellous team. Coming on board were:

- Jenny Wordsworth: I would need someone to be my crew chief to oversee the entire record attempt. When I told my friend Jenny, who I had met through racing, of my intentions to run across America, she immediately offered to help. It was a big commitment to help me plan the record attempt, and to support me from the start to the finish, so I was very grateful to have her involvement for the entire journey.

- Jan Strachan: With everything that needed to be done in mind, a natural choice for one of my crew members was a friend of a friend called Jan. Not only is she a fabulous ultrarunner, she is a member of the Met Police so is well used to sticking to regulations and keeping people in line. She's also an amazing cook. I was delighted when Jan said she would be able to help me for the duration of the world record attempt. She told me she was looking forward to "seeing what went on behind the scenes in a challenge like this and being a part of something incredible." She added that she knew it would be a great opportunity to see America in a way that few people ever experience. I loved her enthusiasm which is another big thing for me when it comes to qualities in a crew member.
- Becky George and her husband, Paul: Becky and I have been friends for years and she has crewed on most of my events, including my John O'Groat's to Land's End (JOGLE) and Ireland world records. In previous challenges, she has always seemed to know what I have needed before I knew it myself – I would tease her saying she must be a witch! She had actually

met Paul thanks to my JOGLE world record, as he was friends with another one of my crew members and had come to visit us one day as we passed through Cornwall. "It was never in any question that I wouldn't want to be part of this!" Becky told me when I rang to ask her if she and Paul would be able to join me in September 2016. This was a massive relief on my part as I couldn't imagine doing it without her.

- Sophie Rooney: Becky and Paul would "only" be able to join me for the first three weeks of the record attempt. When they left, they would be replaced by Sophie, a hugely talented ultrarunner. I hadn't met Sophie in person, but I had heard a lot about her. I was told she was an amazing young woman, mature beyond her 24 years. Being the first woman to run the length of Scandinavia, I knew she would be a great ally as I ran across America, as she would understand exactly what I was going through.

- Fiona Philips, Beccy Williams and Nicola Jones: These are three talented physiotherapists I arranged to have join me at different stages. I knew that running more than 50 miles (80 km) a day for 50 consecutive days would put a huge strain on my body so having a physio on hand every day to provide massage and treatment for my aching muscles would be indispensable.

- My husband, Tim: Trying to run across America without Tim wouldn't have felt right. He is more than just a crucial crew member; he is my husband and my rock. I want to share all the highs and lows of my life with him. Being self-employed, it is difficult for him to take too much time off work as he doesn't get holiday pay, so we agreed he should just join me for a fortnight in the middle of the challenge, flying out at the same time as Sophie.

- Darren Carter: As Tim wouldn't be able to stay for the duration of the run, Jenny recommended Darren, another ultrarunner she knew, to take his place. He would join us for the final weeks of the journey.

It was a relief to have such an experienced and enthusiastic crew in place, making me feel confident and ready to take on the challenge ahead with their full support.

The sponsorship

With my crew lined up and my route planned out, it was time to attract a few sponsors to help make the challenge possible. The amount of money needed to go for a world record of this scale was huge, and although I was happy to put in some of my own money, I certainly couldn't afford to fund it all by myself. Thankfully, my main sponsor James Manclark came on board right at the beginning which gave me a massive boost.

One of the biggest expenses would be the hire of three vehicles for nearly two months. One of these would be an RV which would be home for me and the crew for the duration of the challenge. The other two would be support vehicles driven by the crew. One would leap frog me during the day while I was running, carrying snacks, drinks, ice, spare kit, etc. to give me whenever I met up with them along the way. There would also be a physio in this car in case I needed a quick massage or any other treatment during the day. The other vehicle would be used to scout ahead, checking the route for obstacles, and finding a suitable place for us to park the RV each night (not an easy thing to find as it was 31 ft / 9.45 m long!). The hire of the vehicles alone would cost thousands so I was delighted when VW America offered to be my vehicle sponsors.

Then there was the kit I would need – and plenty of it. Shorts, T-shirts, waterproof jackets, multiple pairs of trainers, lights I could wear when running in the dark, running head torches, fluorescent jackets for me and the crew, tape for strapping my muscles when needed, GPS watches to log my mileage, the list went on and on. I was very grateful when a number of brands agreed to support me.

I am incredibly lucky with the support I receive when I undertake challenges – not only from my friends and family, but also from people I have never met before – so I wanted to try to give something back. I chose two charities I would raise money for during the world record attempt. The first was Marie Curie, a charity close to my heart as they did a wonderful job looking after my father and Tim's brother when they had cancer. The other was Free to Run, for whom I am proud to be an ambassador. They support women and girls who have escaped, or live in, areas of conflict by giving them sporting opportunities. These girls can't just put on their trainers and go for a run like we can, and they are missing out on so much by being deprived of physical activity. Sport teaches us a great deal about ourselves and what we can achieve and gives us a sense of pride, as well as boosting our physical and mental health. The charity has had a massive impact on a lot of the girls by giving them opportunities they wouldn't otherwise have to exercise. I find it is important to know *why* I am taking on a massive challenge when I am running. Raising money for charity is it. I knew that thinking about any donations I would receive for these two worthwhile causes would give me an extra boost to keep going when I hit a rough patch.

A setback in training

While I had been sorting out the logistics, I had also been extremely focused on my training and getting into the best physical shape I could for the September 2016 start date. Over the weeks and months, I gradually began to increase my weekly mileage, clocking up back-to-back long runs ranging from 15–30 miles (24–48 km). My routes would take in quieter roads near my home in Kent, or sometimes I would head off into the forest or local off-road trails to get away from the traffic and give my legs a break from all the Tarmac.

As any endurance athlete knows, there is a fine balance between getting the miles in that you need to do to be fit and prepared for a race, and overdoing it, resulting in injuries and time off training. Unfortunately, around the end of May 2016, the scales tipped the wrong way for me and I started getting a niggle in my right knee that wouldn't go away. I stopped running and saw my osteopath, hoping the rest and some treatment would be all I needed to carry on. But as soon as I started running again, the pain returned and kept getting worse.

One day, I was forced to stop only a few miles in to one of my training runs as my knee hurt so badly. I had to give myself a reality check as I limped home. My knee was taped up so much I looked like an Egyptian mummy, and I was struggling to walk, let alone run. How on earth did I expect to be able to run across America in a couple of months' time? My osteopath suggested I have an MRI scan to see what was going on and unfortunately it was bad news. I had a horizontal lateral tear of the meniscus – a piece of cartilage in the knee that provides cushioning between the thigh bone and shin bone. I was told the tear in my meniscus was bad, and keyhole surgery (an arthroscopy) was the only option. That was the death knell for my run across America starting in the September. I felt completely deflated, frustrated and disappointed when I went home to tell Tim the news.

"The record attempt is off," I told him. "I'm scheduled to have surgery in August, so I'm not even going to be able to run a mile in September, let alone 2,850."

To make it even harder, I had only just announced on social media that I planned on attempting a new world record. Now I would have to tell everyone it wasn't going to happen. After a few days of feeling sorry for myself and wondering if I would have to give up on my dream to run across America completely, I did what I always do and started to look for the positives in my situation. There is always a positive if you look hard enough. I was down but not out.

The surgeon knew of my plan to run across America and he said having the surgery wouldn't prevent me from doing so in the future. It would be best for me to get my knee fixed, give my body time to heal, and then come back stronger. If I followed all the rest and rehab necessary to the letter after the op, I could be ready to start the record attempt in April 2017 instead, I thought. I knew I would struggle at not being able to run in the meantime, but I had to look at the bigger picture and remember what I wanted to achieve. I needed to be in the best possible position to achieve my goal, as I would only have one shot at it. If surgery was what it would take to get me there, I would go under the knife.

I then had to break the disappointing news to my crew and sponsors. I felt terrible for letting them down and asking them to cancel the plans they had put in place in order to come to America in September. Thankfully they were all completely understanding and willing to postpone until I was ready.

I couldn't run while I awaited the day of my operation so I tried to use the time as wisely as I could. I put all my energy into preparing for a running comeback. I did some cycling on an exercise bike at the gym to maintain some fitness (and my sanity!) and did some light weights to strengthen the muscles around my knee. I did lots of research into recovering from knee surgery and asked many of my friends in the ultrarunning community who had been through it for their advice and tips. I was told elite athletes often use underwater treadmills when recovering from injury, as they lessen the impact to the joints. These are expensive pieces of equipment and few and far between so it was unlikely I would be able to find one locally that I would be able to use. I put a call out on Facebook just in case and, as luck would have it, there was an option nearby. It wasn't an underwater treadmill but an anti-gravity one called "Alter G". They look a bit like a bouncy castle surrounding a treadmill and use NASA Differential Air Pressure technology to support your body weight as you run. I discovered there was one at Kent University, and after a few phone calls they kindly agreed to let me use it and support me during my rehab. Knowing I would have the option to train this way when I was ready to run again made me feel so much more positive about my post-op recovery.

Going under the knife

The day of the operation arrived. I felt terrified as Tim took me to the hospital in the morning. No surgery is without risk and I worried about something going wrong. But I reminded myself that if I wanted to achieve my dream of running across America, it had to be done. Having this procedure now was the only way I would have any chance of being able to run 2,850 miles (4,587 km) the following April. When we reached the reception, it was full of other people waiting to be signed in for their various operations. Understandably, they all looked quite miserable and apprehensive, so I tried to smile at them and be relaxed, which wasn't easy as I felt equally nervous about what lay ahead. Eventually we were taken to my room where I was prepared for the op. One surprising and somewhat amusing aspect of this was having to provide the nurse with a urine sample so they could do a pregnancy test.

"There's not much chance of that. I've gone through the menopause!" I told them. She replied they have to test all women pre surgery aged 12 to 65! I was delighted to find out that I wasn't pregnant. I can't imagine how Tim would have reacted had it turned out to be positive!

On my way to the operating theatre I had a good old chat to the anaesthetists who seemed to know all about my running and said they were looking forward to tracking me when I was able to run across America. It was so reassuring to hear there was no negativity about my running considering I was about to have a knee procedure done, and they all believed it would be possible for me to run long distances again. After being pumped full of drugs and attempting to count to ten, the next thing I knew I was waking up in the recovery room feeling great except for a painful throbbing coming from my knee.

When the surgeon came to tell me how well the operation had gone, the first thing I wanted to know, of course, was when I could run again. He said depending on how my knee felt, I might be able to try in around six weeks' time when I had my next check-up. In the meantime, I was encouraged to walk to help keep the knee mobile, and do a series of four exercises two or three times a day to straighten the knee and help get the full range of movement back. I vowed to do these without fail. I was going to do everything I was told to nail my recovery and have a strong knee again. I didn't want to go through all this for nothing.

I counted down the days till the check-up as I was longing to get my trainers back on and head out for a run. When the day finally arrived, I optimistically went to the appointment in my running gear in the hope I could go for a jog afterwards. I was relieved when my surgeon told me he was incredibly impressed with how the joint looked and how it had healed. So, I bravely asked the question he must have known was coming from my attire: "Can I start running again?" I could have given him a massive hug when he replied: "Yes". There were a number of conditions though: it had to be done slowly, I could only run every other day, and I must avoid any big up and down hills. On the days I couldn't run, I was allowed to do some gym work using weights and the cross trainer. I felt extremely lucky that the surgery had gone so well and that I had resisted the urge to run before the check-up. But I wasn't going to wait any longer. Now I had been given the green light, I drove straight from the appointment to the forest where I walked for 10 minutes to warm up, and then ran-walked for a total time of 50 minutes. I can't tell you how good it felt to be outside and running again after 12 weeks of rest pre- and post-surgery. During the run there was no pain in my knee which was an absolute relief, although I did experience some aching afterwards, which the surgeon said may happen as it wouldn't feel normal again for another six to eight weeks.

The rehab

Having my surgeon's permission to run again meant I could start using the Alter G treadmill, so I contacted Kent University to make the arrangements. Deana Stephens, a sports rehabilitator in their sports science department, agreed to assist me with the machine and oversee my rehab. What a stroke of luck. I couldn't have been in better hands as I discovered she had previously worked with rugby players from Saracens and Wasps, and footballers from Gillingham Football Club. When we met, I was delighted to see her hair was dyed my favourite colour, pink – we were definitely going to get along! I felt extremely privileged to be treated by someone of this calibre, as well as having access to some of the best sporting facilities in the country.

My first session began with an assessment of my past history, injuries and current injury as well as discussing my goals. Thankfully Deana didn't fall off her chair when I told her I was planning to run across America the following spring. After assessing my knee, Deana said she was more than happy with the progress and actually felt I was further ahead of my recovery than she thought I would be. All this made me feel a lot happier about the next few weeks ahead. Then it was time to take to the Alter G which was a bizarre experience.

First of all, I had to put on a pair of thick Lycra compression shorts. The treadmill was lowered and I stepped onto it from the back and was then zipped into the bag on it using a zip at the top of the shorts. Deana joked I shouldn't fart at this moment as the smell would remain in the bag until I was unzipped! She then flicked a switch and the bag filled with air around me, gradually lifting me off the floor until I felt as though the shorts were giving me a wedgie. Deana set the machine to take 60 per cent of my body weight. I started out walking for 10 minutes, before being allowed to run for 5 minutes. My arms felt very odd as I had to hold them slightly higher than usual above the bag. I didn't feel the rush of freedom and enjoyment I get from running outside but it still felt good to be doing anything running related, and best of all, there was no pain in my knee. I went home feeling extremely positive and upbeat.

I carried on having rehab sessions with Deana, where we gradually upped the time I spent running on the Alter G treadmill, while reducing the amount of my body weight it took. I carried on cross training in the gym, cycling and doing strengthening exercises for my knee. It was difficult to know how much exercise was too much, or whether I was being too cautious. Occasionally my knee would answer for me by feeling sore and swollen after running. I would also get aches and pains in the muscles surrounding the joint and my hamstrings as they all adapted to me running again. For too long before the op, they had been working harder to compensate for my weak knee. It was like being back at square one again as a runner. I used to be able to run 30 miles (48 km) a day with ease, but by the November, I still couldn't run continuously on the treadmill for more than 3 miles (4.8 km). It is amazing how we take our strength and endurance for granted when we are in peak fitness; we think we're invincible. Coming back from injury was frustrating, humbling, and a much slower process than I had originally anticipated.

It didn't help my mental state that other runners I knew who had knee ops at a similar time to me were already back running long distances and racing. I know we are all different and I shouldn't have compared myself to them, but it was hard not to. There were times when I was walking the dog in the forest and I would think: *I could just run and keep running now for as long as I feel good, nobody would know.* But of course, I would know. Running further than I was supposed to could have delayed my recovery even more, and then I would be kicking myself for my impatience and for not listening to the advice I had been given by the experts.

Added to my frustration was the fact that April was creeping ever closer and I was nowhere near being able to start serious training for the run across America. I started having trouble sleeping as I began waking up at night having panic attacks. I knew I couldn't carry on this way. It dawned on me that I had put extra pressure on my recovery by giving myself a target – especially one so challenging – that was only months away. It wasn't good for my mental or physical health. I had to take a step back and stop pushing myself so hard.

At the beginning of January 2017, I decided to voice my fears to Deana to see what she thought. "I'm starting to think attempting the world record in April is too soon," I told her. "I feel as though I'm trying to rush everything, and it would be better to postpone it again to take the pressure off."

"I completely agree with you," she said with a sigh of relief. We agreed that waiting till September, a whole year after my surgery, would be much more realistic.

From that moment, I felt like a weight had been lifted from my shoulders. I should have postponed it to the

September instead of the April in the first place, but I had underestimated how slow my recovery would be, and how long it would take for me to be able to build my mileage back up. For the next few months, I was finally able to do just that. I was able to leave the Alter G treadmill behind and hit the roads and trails for longer distances again. It was a joy to be running outside, even though it was winter and the weather was often freezing cold and wet. I carried on doing rehab exercises in the gym every week. This is something I had previously always neglected in my training as I find it so dull. But now I saw how hugely beneficial it could be to my strength and running gait. I would do repetitions of squats, calf raises, leg presses, glute bridges, "monster walks" and the clam to name just a few.

On the subject of my running gait, this was something I wanted to work on as my knee does have a habit of rolling inwards, which is likely to have contributed to my problems in the first place. I went to StrideUK in Hove where their enthusiastic and knowledgeable team took good care of me. Before my running style was filmed and analysed as I ran on the treadmill – first in trainers, then barefoot – I had lines drawn on the back of my legs. When I ran, I had to try to keep my body within the middle section of targets on the wall in front of the machine. I then had to turn and run in the other direction so they could gain a full picture of how my biomechanics work. I only had to run for about 10 minutes to provide them with a wealth of information about my weird and wonderful running style.

Watching the footage on the computer, lines could be drawn from my hip down to my foot, showing how much my knees go inwards as I land each stride. I was concerned they would recommend I work on completely changing my running gait and cadence – something that takes a lot of time and perseverance – but Mitch, who was doing the analysis, told me my running gait had helped me achieve all my previous endurance feats, so it obviously worked pretty well. There was no point trying to change how I ran, but what I could do is work on strengthening certain muscle groups to support the knees and stop them rolling in quite as much.

It turned out that my quads (in the thigh) were the dominant muscles in my legs, which meant I needed to do more exercises to activate my glute muscles (in the bottom). I also had a slight forward tilt – again this was mainly to do with my strong quads – and could be amended by doing certain exercises and drills regularly. The result would be I should be able to run faster and more efficiently – and be less prone to injury. All of which would be hugely beneficial to my world record attempt, which was now just seven months away. They say knowledge is power, and gaining all this extra information about how my body worked definitely made me feel as though I could become a running powerhouse again. No stone was being left unturned in my quest to prepare myself to run across America.

Back on track

By June 2017, I was noticing the positive effects of doing all the strengthening exercises and drills, and I was back to following a training schedule set for me by my coach Ray Zahab. I first met Ray when we both ran Badwater in 2005 (an infamous 135-mile / 217-km race in the USA, starting at Badwater Basin in Death Valley and finishing in the portals of Mount Whitney). We then met again in 2006 at the Libyan Challenge, a gruelling ultramarathon that he won. In addition to being a talented ultrarunner, he's a Canadian adventurer and founder of Impossible2Possible, an adventure-based learning programme that takes young people on educational and character-forming expeditions.

As well as being a friend, he's the perfect coach for me and I completely trust his methods and training plans. He advised me not to do any races before the America world record attempt and just focus on the training. After building up my long runs gradually, I was back to doing up to 30 miles (48 km) two to three times a week, and up to 12–15 miles (19–24 km) twice a week. At times friends were able to join me, which was wonderful as it can get incredibly boring running these long distances alone – although I knew I shouldn't complain about it and just be grateful that I could run again after everything I had been through in the past year.

Some days the enormity of what I was taking on was overwhelming and I would feel a wave of panic moving up inside me. It wasn't just the fact that I was taking on this huge challenge, but that I would be doing it with all the eyes of the ultrarunning community and beyond on me. The expectation and the attention was an added pressure. Then to pile the pressure on even more, I found out that another ultrarunner, Sandra Villines, was also planning to go for the world record, and, like me, she would be starting her run in September.

I didn't know much about Sandra other than that she was American and had been the first female at Badwater in 2017. As far as I was aware, she wasn't known for doing multi-day events. I learnt that she would be setting off a few days after me, which was a relief, as I felt I could focus more on myself if I wasn't chasing her. There was no chance we would cross paths as she was going to do a completely different route from San Francisco to New York. She would be following the route used by Pete Kostelnick when he set the male record for the fastest time to run across America. I knew I shouldn't worry about what Sandra was doing. I had my plan and she had hers. But the fact we would both be running at the same time created more pressure that I could have done without. Now it wasn't just a world record attempt, it was a race, which gave it a different dynamic.

Mental battles

I started to have meltdowns at night-time when my mind was racing, thinking about what I still needed to do and worrying about all the things that could go wrong. After finally getting to sleep, my troubles would always seem smaller and more surmountable in the morning. But one day when I was midway through a 25-mile (40-km) run, I felt huge a panic attack coming on. As I kept thinking about how far 2,850 miles (4,587 km) is to run, my heart rate started spiking and I felt as though I couldn't breathe. Negative thoughts kept popping up in my mind: *I can't do this. It is too much. Whose idea was it to run across America anyway? It is impossible. I have to give up.* I stopped my watch and sat in a field where I promptly burst into tears.

When I had calmed down and regained my composure, I gave myself a good talking to. This was MY idea. It was something I was passionate about. The pressure and expectation were all of my own making, and were part and parcel of what goes into attempting a world record.

STOP moaning and get on with it, I thought. *In America it is going to be so much worse. I will be covering large distances each day and feeling exhausted, but if I want this record I have to keep going.*

I stood up, took a deep breath, restarted my watch and resumed running, replacing my negative thoughts with positive ones. I started visualizing the amazing scenery I would see when I ran across America, as well as the people

I would meet. I thought about the many marvellous people who had put their faith in me, from those who had aided my comeback from the knee op, to the crew who were ready and waiting to join me on the journey. I didn't want to let anyone down, so I had to put in the effort now to be totally physically and mentally prepared. I also thought about the emotions I would experience and how it would all be worth it as I ran over the George Washington Bridge into Manhattan and then up the steps of New York City Hall to set a new world record. I could just imagine what a fantastic feeling that would be. By the end of the run, I was feeling much more upbeat and back to my usual positive self.

However, there were other days when my resolve wasn't so strong, and occasionally I would end up cutting a training run short by a mile or two. On those days I would return home feeling as though I had let myself down by giving in too easily, but also knowing I had no more to give.

"There are always going to be days when things don't go to plan, and this is one of those days," Tim wisely told me after one such run when I was beating myself up about those missed miles. He then added with concern: "Have a rest and something to eat now, you look like you are losing too much weight."

In the past, I would have taken such a comment as a compliment and felt a huge sense of achievement about my weight loss. But having recovered from an eating disorder that had made me frail, weak and facing hospitalization in my twenties, I knew I couldn't afford to become dangerously thin again.

Taking up ultrarunning had been a key aspect of my recovery, as I discovered that if I wanted to run long distances, I had to eat more to fuel my training. I didn't want to fail in America because I couldn't sustain my energy levels. I thought I had been eating enough, but with all the extra miles I was putting in, I obviously needed more. It was good I had Tim to support me as I can still suffer from body dysmorphia when I see myself in the mirror. I also had no idea what I weighed, because I haven't owned any scales since I was 30. I find they are too detrimental to my health as I become fixated on the numbers they reveal.

At the height of my eating disorder, I was weighing myself multiple times a day to check if I had put any weight on. Once on the scales, if I found my weight had gone down, I would feel ecstatic. If it went up, I would feel disgusted with myself and vow not to eat again until it had dropped. I never want to go back to that time but being on scales always seems to trigger those emotions, even now, decades on. For example, a couple of years ago a doctor who I don't usually see wanted to know my weight when I had a check-up. My usual doctors know I will close my eyes when I stand on the scales and ask not to know the result, but this one didn't and told me my weight. The impact on me was instant and left me in turmoil for the rest of the day. Knowing what I weighed made me instinctively want to diet, but the rational part of my brain knew that wasn't sensible. My mood was low and I felt terrible about my body image. All thanks to standing on those scales.

When Tim expressed his concern, I thought perhaps I should brave the scales again to find out what my weight was. I psyched myself up and stepped onto a set at the gym the next day. This was a big mistake. Once again, those old feelings came rushing back. When I saw what I weighed, I felt happy and accomplished. I was thin and this was the proof! I was sucked back in and on my next visit to the gym a few days later, I weighed myself again. Result! I had lost a few more pounds! Seeing the reading on the scales drop felt delightful and I was on a high as I stepped off; I had achieved my goal of losing weight. But then I realized this wasn't my goal any more. I didn't want to lose weight. In fact, I would be better off putting it on if I wanted to be able to keep up my training and then be strong enough to run across America.

Suddenly, I felt angry with myself that after all these years, my state of mind could still so easily be governed by my weight.

I'm definitely not going back on the scales again, I vowed. I knew if I did, it would become a competition to see how many pounds I could lose each week, and I would lose sight of my running ambitions.

Getting the right nutrition

I had to stay focused on the US run, and that meant making a conscious effort to eat more during and after a run, and not worrying about what I weighed as a result. Eating during my long training runs is something I have always found difficult, as I just don't get hungry. Whatever I take with me I don't feel like eating, so I end up not bothering. Finding foods that complement you while running is very personal, and what works for one person might make another feel heavy-stomached and nauseous.

I know bananas are a popular choice with others as they provide excellent energy and are easy to eat and digest on the move, but I find they go brown and mushy from all the bouncing up and down in my pack – not at all appealing or appetising.

When I ran across America, I would be burning more than 6,000 calories a day. The crew would prepare three nutritious meals a day for me to eat when I wasn't running but this still wouldn't be enough. I would also need to eat plenty of snacks in between or I would soon run out of energy. I started using my training runs to experiment with food I could eat on the go. This was both practice for when and what I would eat running across America, and fuel to get me through the training. I found one of the best snacks for me were flapjacks with added chia seeds. Marmite, peanut butter and jam sandwiches cut into fingers were also easy to grab and eat while running. For hydration, I tried taking coconut water as it is known as a natural electrolyte drink because of its vitamin and mineral content, but I disliked the taste so I stuck to water or a weak orange squash.

To ensure further that I would be eating enough in America, when Jan first agreed to join the crew, I asked her if she was willing to be my "head chef". I knew Jan was an excellent cook who had crewed at races before, so she had a few tried and tested dishes up her sleeve. I was conscious it was a big responsibility to place on her shoulders. It meant Jan would be doing the majority of the cooking and meal planning for the crew and me. She would need to ensure the meals and snacks she provided would give me enough calories and nutrients to fuel my running and aid my recovery. To help her, I put her in touch with an experienced sport nutritionist who was able to provide a recommended eating plan for a multi-day ultrarunner that Jan could use as a guide. I was so grateful to Jan for taking this on as it was another weight off my mind knowing my nutritional needs were covered.

The final countdown

When I wasn't running or spending time with my family, I was putting the other final details in place for the run across America. Head of crew Jenny and I had video calls on a regular basis to discuss the plans and go over and over the daily routine. She then put together an information pack to give to all the other crew members so everyone would be up to speed with the schedule and each day should run like clockwork. We couldn't afford to waste time when the challenge started with any faffing or confusion, so it was important to get everything and everyone organized in advance. Meanwhile, Jan researched and put together a list of supermarkets along the way to ensure we would always be stocked up with supplies, especially as some parts of the route would be quite remote.

When the day came to turn my calendar over to September 2017, I felt a rush of panic and excitement. In a few days' time, I would be boarding a flight to America, and then starting to run across the third largest continent in the world a few days after that. Immediately my mind started racing with what still needed to be done. I realized that until we arrived in L.A. there wasn't actually much more I could do. The training was done, the flights had been booked, the vehicles were arranged, the route was finalized. It seemed there was nothing I hadn't thought of to ensure I was fully prepared for what lay ahead. I knew I was as ready as I would ever be. It was finally time for my American dream to become a reality.

CHAPTER TWO

THE ADVENTURE BEGINS

I landed in L.A. along with Becky, Paul and Jan on 3 September with masses of kit. Luckily, we had managed to get it onto the plane without having to pay any excess baggage. Jenny (who would be joining us in a couple of days) had instructed everyone to bring only one piece of luggage as space was going to be tight in the RV, but however hard I tried, I simply couldn't fit all my kit into one large bag so I ended up with three! On arrival at the airport, our first job was to collect the two support cars provided by VW America that the crew would use. We dubbed them "Penelope" and "Tiggy".

Once we had collected the cars – which had been decked out with all the logos of my sponsors – we drove into the city to spend a couple of nights in a hotel. I had factored in these days to give me time to recover from the long-haul flight and adjust to the new time zone. I knew how tired and fatigued I would be once the run began so I could do without jetlag as well. When I wasn't putting my feet up, we headed out to the Hollywood Hills to see the famous sign, but I wasn't really in the right frame of mind for sightseeing with the world record attempt just around the corner. I took everyone to City Hall where we walked the first section of the route. This put my mind at rest about which direction I would be running in when I started – imagine if I had gone the wrong way minutes into the run! It sounds silly as I had been there before and knew exactly which way to go, but it made me feel better and was one less thing to worry about.

A couple of days before the record attempt began there was still lots to be done. Jan and I went back to the airport to pick up Jenny. We then all drove to a big Walmart supermarket to stock up on supplies; I don't think I have ever been to such a huge shop. I'm sure you could have fitted several football pitches inside. Armed with a list as long as your arm, we filled three trolleys as we made our way around the massive store; the whole process took about 3 hours. I knew we would need a lot of food to feed six people but paying the bill was a bit of a shock! The day finished with my main sponsor and friend James Manclark and his wife, Patricia, taking the team out for dinner which was wonderful. They had flown out to L.A. especially so they could be at the start and wave me off.

With one day to go, my nerves were really starting to kick in big time and there was still lots to be done. After breakfast, the crew had a meeting to go through everything. Becky, who knows me best, gave everyone an insight into how I work as a runner so they knew what to expect and how best to help me. Then it was time to collect the RV which would be our home for the duration of the challenge. The RV, which we fondly dubbed Monty, was a massive 31 feet (9.45 m) long – with extending sides when parked. I didn't appreciate quite how huge it was until I saw it. Stepping inside to explore it for the first time was extremely exciting. There was a double bedroom for me at the back, two slide-out bunk beds, a double bed above the driver's seat, and two single beds, providing enough space to sleep eight people. There was one small shower room for everyone to share and a kitchen with all mod cons including a microwave, small fridge and an oven. I was delighted I would have my own space to retreat to every night on my journey and extremely grateful that I wasn't going to be the one to have to drive it!

Once back at our hotel, with all our luggage and supplies to pack on board the RV, the crew spent most of the rest of the day organizing the kit and food, deciding where it should go so it would be easily accessible when required. With all of us set to live in a confined space for the next couple of months, it was extremely important it was kept clean and tidy, with a place for everything, and everything in its place. I let them get on with it so I could rest and be out of their way. There was no need for me to know where everything was kept since I wouldn't be doing any of the cooking or washing up (lucky me!). From now on, I just wanted to focus on the running and let my crew take care of everything else.

After having a takeaway pizza for supper, our final crew member Fiona arrived and gave me a massage before I settled down for my last night in a comfortable hotel bed. The crew stayed up till after midnight trying to sort out the RV until Jenny quite rightly sent them to bed. It was a relief to know everyone was getting along and working well together given most of them had only just met.

I had a quick check of my messages from home before going to sleep as I thought I had better make the most of the hotel Wi-Fi. It would be difficult to get a signal once we were off the beaten track, and I knew once we got going I wouldn't always have the energy, or the inclination, to read them. During the run, I would leave all the social media updates on my accounts to my crew as this was definitely something I didn't want to spend time on. My job was to run. When I checked my emails that evening, I had received a wonderful message from two amazing women who I had been in touch with a few years before. They had asked me for some advice on tackling their first multi-day ultra. Wishing me luck, they told me to remember the tips I had given them: "There will be moments when you feel like you can't go on. Take five minutes, sort yourself out, and remember your body is capable of doing a lot more than you think it can. Remember the reason you are running this race, focus on finishing one day at a time. If that's too much, focus on checkpoint to checkpoint but keep moving forward."

I knew I needed to heed my own advice as the nerves were starting to kick in, and like we all do before races, I was wondering: *Have I done enough training? Will I be able to do this?*

As I tried to nod off to sleep, I still couldn't quite believe where I was and what I was about to do. I don't normally sleep well before a big event because I am so nervous, as well as excited, so I didn't expect this night to be any different.

In the morning, I will be starting the longest run I have ever attempted, I thought. I could picture the route map across America in my mind. It was a LONG way. Had I finally bitten off more than I could chew? Was I going to be up to this epic challenge? I was about to find out.

7–11 SEPTEMBER
STATE ONE: CALIFORNIA
DISTANCE COVERED: 279.36 MILES (449.59 KM)
L.A. CITY HALL TO US-95, SOUTH OF PALM GARDENS, CALIFORNIA
(Locations are approximate as we often crossed the state lines in remote areas)

I woke before my alarm went off at 4 a.m.

This is it, I thought as I got out of bed to have breakfast and a large cup of coffee. *The big day has finally arrived.* After all the worrying, self-doubt and panic attacks that had gone before, I felt strangely calm. It was show time. Nothing left to do now but run. We drove to City Hall where I would start running at 6 a.m. on the dot. When we arrived, there were loads of trucks and people milling around. They weren't there for me but were part of a film crew who were setting up to start filming scenes at the Hall a few hours later. It all added to the buzz of excitement.

There were a number of dignitaries present who had come to be my official starters, and I was surprised to see a piper on the steps. Carol from Scrumptious Productions, who is Scottish like me, had organized for him to send me off by playing my favourite tune, "Highland Cathedral". *How lovely*, I thought. She, and her colleague Susie Wright, had been at City Hall bright and early to film the start of my journey and were ready to follow us the whole way in their own RV. I was also touched to have James and Patricia there to wave me off as promised. I greeted everyone with a big smile and hugs and then it was time to get going. I took a deep breath as the gathered crowd gave me a 10-second countdown.

"Three, two, one... GO!"

I was off, taking my first step of many towards New York. There was no going back now. I had been building up to this point for so long and now here I was, finally starting my run across America.

It felt such a relief to be on my way. All that time planning and training came down to this. Becky ran with me for the first 11 miles (17.7 km) and we were both buoyant. I was so glad she was with me to start the journey as it was nice to have a close friend to share the experience with. I don't know if it was down to all the adrenaline and nerves in my system, or because of the relief I felt at finally being on the road, but I was flying and I felt fabulous. I went off "like the clappers," as one observer of my Strava stats later put it, and perhaps I was going a little too fast. I knew from my previous experiences of running long distances that it is crucial to rein it in, especially on the first few days when you feel great, or you will pay for it later. It wasn't my intention to be running quickly but I decided not to look at the pace on my watch and just go by feel. I found out later that, at times, the average pace I had been doing was around 10 minutes per mile (6 minutes 12 seconds per km). This pace might not be fast to some, but given I still had to run thousands of miles over more than 50 consecutive days, it was a little speedy.

We were running on the pavements through L.A. which wasn't too bad to begin with, but as the day wore on and the city came to life, it was hard to get into a rhythm as there were people everywhere. There were lots of roads to cross and sometimes I found myself waiting for what seemed like forever for the lights to change. This was quite frustrating as all I could think about was the time I was wasting standing around. We knew it would be like this, which is why I had always planned to run 60 miles (96.5 km) on the first day.

L.A. is so incredibly spread out, I would need to run that far to reach the outer city limits, so that the following day's run would then be on the quieter open roads.

Once Becky stopped running with me, I didn't need to worry about getting lost as the roads out of L.A. are pretty straight. But just in case, I had downloaded the route onto my trusty Garmin (a GPS watch), which became my safety blanket. As I ran further and further from the city centre and more into suburbia, the temperature soared to around 38°C (100°F), which was a bit of a shock coming from the UK. Although I love warm weather, I started to feel as though I was going to overheat. To my relief, I noticed one of the houses ahead had a sprinkler going in their front garden. It was like seeing an oasis in the desert. I politely asked the owners, who were standing chatting by their door, if they would mind if I stood underneath it to cool down. I think they thought I was totally mad but nevertheless said yes and watched in amusement as I revelled in the cool shower. It was heaven!

By the afternoon, the heat was getting to me even more and I was having trouble keeping any food down as I ate on the run. Each time I tried, a horrid gag reflex would make me vomit. It was a relief finally to reach my stop for the night after 61.4 miles (98.8 km) of running. I was so happy to climb into the RV, knowing that once inside I could have another cool shower and eat some food while not running so I wouldn't feel sick. Jan served up the most delicious pasta dish followed by cake and ice cream. I'm not someone who usually eats pudding but after running such a long way, my body was in need of the extra calories.

The crew had spent all day organizing the RV and getting my stuff unpacked for me. Becky talked me through the drawers and cupboards in my room letting me know exactly where I could find everything. I felt so grateful that they had been very busy making sure everything was in order and as easy as possible for me. It felt fantastic to have the first day under my belt. Running across America was now my reality. I wasn't dreaming; the adventure had truly begun.

* * *

It was a relief to wake up on day two with my legs feeling great. I was raring to get going again, even though I hadn't slept well and had bags under my eyes that I could fit a weekly supermarket shop into! Having left the city I was looking forward to running through the Morongo Indian Reservation which is set at the foot of the beautiful San Gorgonio and San Jacinto mountains and spans more than 35,000 acres. The scenery there was just beautiful. The mountains towered on all sides under an enormous blue sky; even the giant cloud formations had a beauty all of their own. It is one of nine reservations that were created by President Ulysses S. Grant in 1876 and remains home to the Morongo Band of Mission Indians today. They created an amazing business opportunity when they opened a bingo hall there in 1983 that went on to become one of the most successful Indian gaming facilities in California. They then opened the luxurious Morongo Casino, Resort and Spa in 2004. I would have loved to stop off there for some R&R but unfortunately on this trip there was no time for such luxuries!

We discovered my route would pass through the reservation when we did the recce in May 2016. It proved quite a headache as I needed to gain permission to run through it, as any alternative options were too long and complicated. After months of emailing backwards and forwards, I was eventually given the go-ahead on one condition: I had to be accompanied by a police escort. When I reached the entrance to the reservation the police were waiting for us by the security checkpoint. Jan, who would be running through it with me, started chatting to them about how she was also a police officer and this instantly broke the ice. It came in handy throughout the challenge when we were regularly stopped by local law enforcement wondering what we were up to. Jan would show her warrant card (badge) to them and share experiences about what it was like to be a police officer. She had also brought a supply of little New Scotland Yard pin badges which she gave out, and was pleased to acquire a selection of badges from the officers we met along the way in return.

As a serving police officer, it hadn't been easy for Jan to get such a long time off work (nine weeks in total) to be part of my crew. She had to gain permission from her Chief Superintendent, who thankfully saw it was a trip and adventure of a lifetime and supported her application. In return, Jan had to work numerous weekends to make up her shifts, and ensure her team were supported while she was away. I was so grateful to her for doing this.

Once we'd had a nice chat outside the reservation with our escorts, the barrier was raised to allow us all to pass. I ran with the police car moving slowly ahead of me with the blue lights flashing but sirens off. I felt like a film star! It made the journey so much easier as the police would hold up the traffic when we reached crossroads, allowing me to keep going without having to stop till it was safe to cross. I was sad to leave them behind when we reached the boundary of the reservation a couple of hours later. Jan and I agreed it had been a privilege to be able to run through it. The views of the mountains around us as we ran through the desert-like land had been incredible. It was something neither of us would ever forget.

As I carried on running, the terrain couldn't have been more different from the day before: we were now off-road and it really felt as though we were in the middle of nowhere. It was a relief to be away from the crowded pavements, traffic and buildings in this largely untouched part of California, but it was very hilly. Jan was still running with me to keep me company though she soon started to struggle as the temperature kept rising.

"It's so hot!" Jan exclaimed after a few miles, as she wiped sweat from her brow. "Are you feeling OK?" she asked me.

She was amazed when I told her I felt fine. After the previous day running in the heat, I already felt acclimatized and I just kept telling myself I had run in far hotter temperatures before, when racing across deserts and through Death Valley during the Badwater Ultramarathon.

If I could do it then, I can do it now, I told myself. Also, I knew I had no choice but to grin and bear it. I couldn't afford to stop and have a break. Jan could though, so I urged her to cool off in the air-conditioned support car at the next meeting point. She was soon relieved to see Jenny and Fiona ahead waiting for us and I checked she was OK before I carried on running.

"I'm sorry," she said as she took refuge from the heat in the cool car. "It is supposed to be me looking after you, not the other way around!"

I didn't mind though as I didn't want any of the crew to suffer on my account. I needed them to stay happy and healthy. I couldn't cool off in the air-conditioned car but the crew had another idea to help me. They handed me a headband filled with some ice cubes which I wrapped around my wrist, but first I took out one of the ice-cubes to suck. My mouth had been incredibly dry all morning, and no matter how much I drank, I simply couldn't quench my thirst. What a relief it was to have something cold in my mouth.

I carried on alone and realized at the next stop-off I would have to eat more than just ice cubes. I felt repulsed at the thought. The heat and the mileage I was doing was really suppressing my appetite and I just wasn't enjoying eating. I had already made this very clear to the crew. They had been putting up with my moaning every time they handed me a snack. I often ungratefully refused to eat whatever they had first prepared in favour of something else. I knew this wasn't fair as the crew – particularly Jan – had done a fantastic job of meal and snack planning to ensure I would have delicious food that would give me all the calories I needed. But even though they were preparing tasty snacks and had planned to give me plenty of variety to stop me from getting bored eating the same things day after day, I was still often reluctant to eat what they provided. Jan said she sympathized as she had experienced a loss of appetite when she had done ultra races in the past, but she wasn't going to let me off.

"I'm going to have to insist you eat even if you don't want to," she told me at our next meet-up, handing over a wrap she had prepared. She won this tense stand-off as I did reluctantly eat it, but I am embarrassed to say I wasn't at all appreciative of the effort she had made to make it. I ate the food because I had to, but it was a real chore. As I ran the next stint, I thought: *The crew must be dreading seeing me every time I arrive at the support car knowing how grumpy I am being about food.* I decided I had to stop moaning as it wasn't fair on them and it was such a negative thing to do. I needed to eat to run so I just had to get down whatever was offered to me without complaint. I told myself that from here on in, I would not complain every time I had to eat.

The following day saw a change in the weather as the hot sunshine was replaced by heavy rain, thunder and lightning. It was one extreme to the other, and to make it even harder, the next 5 miles (8 kilometres) I had to run were uphill. After running cross-country the day before, it was lovely to be back on a road. However, because of the heavy downfall there were flash floods, turning the road very quickly into a river. My feet were soon soaking wet through, and to make it even worse, when cars drove past, they would spray me with even more water from the puddles. I dreaded a big lorry passing as that meant another drenching. It reminded me of the ice bucket challenge that happened in 2014 when you had a bucket of cold water thrown over you!

When doing my research, I had learnt that flash floods often happened in this area. Flash flood was such an accurate term for it as the roads would go from dry to flooded in the blink of an eye. If it got too bad, roads had to be closed by the police. I hoped that wouldn't happen today as it would mean finding an alternative route, taking up valuable time. Running with wet shoes and slightly swollen feet had caused two small blisters to rub on the inside of each of my feet, giving me a most unwelcome stinging pain. Apart from that soreness, my body had been holding up really well, so

I wanted them to heal as quickly as possible to alleviate my discomfort.

Once I finished for the day, I washed my feet and let the blisters dry out overnight. The following morning, Fiona covered them up with moleskin plasters to prevent them rubbing again. It worked a treat and they soon disappeared, but I kept putting the moleskin plasters on every day just in case. Susie from the film crew was amazed at how quickly the blisters healed and how I dealt with the discomfort in the meantime, having been unfortunate enough to see the state of my feet when filming me in the RV the evening they were at their worst. "You're like Wolverine from the X-Men!" she joked when she saw how quickly they healed.

Thankfully the rain eased off and the rest of the week became warmer and brighter again which meant I was able to enjoy running on the outskirts of the famous Joshua Tree National Park. This is a vast protected area in southern California, characterized by rugged rock formations, stark desert landscapes and named after the region's twisted, bristled Joshua trees.

A resounding memory of running through California was always looking up and marvelling at how big the sky was above me. I loved running during the sunrise each morning as the huge blue sky became filled with streaks of pink as the sun rose above the earth. There is nothing more peaceful or beautiful than witnessing the start of a new day.

I needed such pick-me-ups as I ploughed on through California, heading further along the iconic Route 66, which spans 2,400 miles (3,862 km) from Chicago, Illinois, to Santa Monica, California. The magnificent mountains and lush terrain I had run through before gave way to much bleaker terrain. Now I was mostly running across wide open desert with salt flats for mile after mile. These salt flats looked rather brown and dirty, not like the glimmering white ones I saw in Death Valley while taking part in the Badwater Ultramarathon.

Among the other highlights of running through California were the people I met along the way. One was a lovely lady who had been following me via my tracker on the website. She decided to come and cheer me on as I was passing very close to where she lived. She had made a sign to wish me good luck and I burst into tears when I saw her beaming and waving her "Go Mimi" placard by the roadside. After a quick chat and a hug, the opportunist crew got her to sign one of the witness statement forms as I headed off down the road again.

At another point, as I approached a railway crossing on Route 66, the lights started flashing, indicating a train was coming, so I had to stop. I knew this could be a long wait. Everything I had seen so far in America was so much larger than I had ever seen anywhere else, and that is especially true of the trains. They are absolutely enormous. Becky and Jan counted one that was more than 100 containers in length and two containers high. They were quite amazing to see whizzing though the landscape when I was running along, and the drivers would always toot at me. But they did cause long delays whenever I was waiting to cross a line as container after container shot by. At this particular stop, I got chatting to a young couple in the car waiting beside me and they couldn't believe the journey I was on. They signed a witness statement form and then gave me a high five when I was on my way. "You go girl, you've got this!" they told me.

I then passed the famous Roy's Cafe in the Mojave Desert town of Amboy, which has been featured in numerous films and pop videos. It first opened as a petrol station in 1938 for travellers on Route 66. In its heyday it became a successful cafe and motel, and was a renowned stopping point for people on road trips, its neon sign beaming in the distance as they approached.

The opening of California's Interstate 40 led to a huge loss of business and it went into decline over a number of years. It was revived to its former glory in 2008 and now attracts people like me passing through on Route 66 adventures. When I ran past, I was greeted with loud cheers of encouragement from the people outside including a group of bikers from Finland. They later passed by as they continued their journey, waving and cheering, before stopping further up the road to have their photos taken with me. I cherished moments like these. It was always such a boost to be given support and encouragement from people who I had never met before.

The last few miles of each day were always the hardest, especially if there wasn't any beautiful scenery to look at. Any of my crew who ran with me at the end of the day would sometimes have to put up with me grumbling. I would be particularly grumpy if the end point had to be further on than originally planned, due to being unable to find a safe place to park the RV for the night. It was silly of me to get frustrated about it as ultimately I had to do these miles – doing extra one day would mean doing fewer on another – but often by the end of each day I was just desperate to stop and rest.

"Just a little bit further," the crew would say to me to cushion the blow, as sometimes it would actually be a few miles more than planned until I reached the RV. Then I would become like a frustrated child on a car journey wailing "are we nearly there yet?" I always prefer to know exactly how far I have to go when I'm running.

The other alternative if there wasn't somewhere to park on the route was for me to run the intended distance for that day, and then "stake out". I would then be driven to where the RV had been able to park, and back the following day to the exact point on the route where I had stopped in order to continue running. This was all officially videoed and documented for Guinness.

Occasionally Carol and Susie would park their RV elsewhere, as it was hard enough to find an ideal spot to park one large vehicle overnight, let alone two. They told me they were constantly struck by how generous people were, allowing them to park on their land and use their washing machines to do their laundry, despite the fact they were complete strangers.

"Everyone we have met has been really fascinated by what you're doing," Susie told me. "The most common question we are asked about your run is 'why?'" She then observed: "People have been so kind and incredibly welcoming in a way that had the situation been reversed – had it been an American running through Britain – I just can't see people opening up their homes and land in the same way."

By now, the crew and I were in a routine that was working well. Every evening, they would plan for the day ahead after I had gone to bed, writing out the schedule on a big whiteboard we had taken with us. This included the times I would aim to arrive at our proposed lunch stop, when I would resume running again afterwards, and my target miles for that day. When Tim and Sophie arrived weeks later, they would always draw a little mouse, who would be doing something different each day, alongside the stats. I always looked forward to seeing what they had come up with when I looked at the board.

We had agreed in advance that our day would always start at 4.30 a.m. I am a morning person and I have found when doing previous multi-day running challenges that it is best for me to run earlier in the day, rather than later into the evening. The latter would involve running in the dark for longer and I always felt more tired as the day went on.

I would dress while eating breakfast and start running by 5 a.m. Becky would usually run the first miles of the day with me, which we would spend warming up and settling into a comfortable pace, chatting about all sorts. I was touched when Becky told me she felt incredibly privileged to be part of my adventure and sharing this time with me. I felt the same, especially as she and Paul were actually on their honeymoon! They tied the knot in May 2016, and decided to postpone their honeymoon so they could use the extended time off work to join me in America. We joked it was their "runningmoon". I was so grateful they were willing to do this. They were both well aware before it started that it wouldn't be a relaxing holiday as there would be a lot of work to do every day. Plus, they would be sharing it with me and a number of other crew members they hadn't met before – not your typical honeymoon!

Once Becky stopped running with me in the mornings, I would carry on alone, or with another member of the crew joining me for short periods, until I reached approximately 30–32 miles (48–51.5 km). This would be followed by a 20–30-minute lunch break, usually around midday, leaving 25–28 miles (40–45 km) to run in the afternoon to complete my daily target mileage. I preferred running the longer stint first as psychologically it made me feel much more positive. In the morning I would count up the miles; in the afternoon, I would count them down. Once the target mileage had been achieved, I would stop my watches and hand them to

Jenny together with the tracker to be charged, before going into the RV. I would shower if I had the energy, or just have a quick wash if not. I would then have a massage, usually while eating an evening meal lovingly cooked by Jan or another member of the crew. I would eat the main course while the fronts of my legs were being massaged, then flip over and eat dessert while the backs of my legs were rubbed. Finally, Fiona would rub some Cowshed foot balm into my feet which was soothing and relaxing and I would go to bed as quickly as possible in order to get as much rest as I could. Every night before heading to my bed I always remembered to say thank you to the crew for all the hard work they had done; it's a small phrase but an extremely important one.

On day five, things didn't quite go to plan. I left the RV as usual at 5 a.m. but stupidly forgot to take my inhaler. I usually carried it – and water bottles – in a running vest I wore with pockets and pouches. I was diagnosed with asthma at the age of eight and I always carry my inhaler when I'm running, just in case I need it. Occasionally I can become breathless when running in cold and wet conditions, and traffic fumes can trigger my asthma as well.

Typically, this was one of those days I was beside a busy road and the fumes were getting to me. I was finding breathing more difficult than usual. We had arranged to meet Jenny and Fiona in the support vehicle after I had run 4 miles (6.4 km) but Jan didn't think I should try to keep running that far without my inhaler. We had only gone half a mile at this point, so she ran back to Monty to get it, along with my water bottle, which I had also forgotten – I must have been very keen to get running that day! It was just as well Jan went back as there was no sign of Jenny and Fiona in Penelope when we reached the 4-mile mark where we had arranged to meet them.

"Where are they?" I asked Jan with concern. As well as being worried about them, it was another baking hot day and I had drunk all the water Jan had gone back for earlier. I really needed a fresh supply from them.

"There's no sign of them at all," Jan said scanning the road in all directions. "I can't phone either as I don't have a signal." We had no choice but to carry on and hope to see them sooner rather than later. They eventually caught up with us a few miles later looking extremely distraught.

"We're so sorry for the delay!" said Jenny as she leapt out of the vehicle. "The car got stuck in the sand and we couldn't move!"

The quick-thinking and resourceful pair had ended up using foot mats and a chopping board from the RV to get themselves out. They were the best items they had to hand to wedge under the wheels to give them enough traction to free the car from the sand. I was just glad they were OK and I carried on running without delay. It obviously wasn't Jenny's day, as she was then stung by a scorpion which I believe had crept into her shoe before she put it on. We were all concerned about the effects of the poison as she started to feel a little tired and feverish. As we were in the middle of nowhere, she couldn't get to a hospital right away. Luckily her partner is a doctor, so she called him for some advice. He told her what to do and the signs to look out for in case of an adverse reaction. Thankfully she soon felt better, and we could turn our attention to an exciting afternoon ahead where I would be crossing over into my second state of Nevada, shortly followed by my third, Arizona.

11 SEPTEMBER
STATE TWO: NEVADA
DISTANCE COVERED: 21.23 MILES (34.17 KM)
SOUTH OF PALM GARDENS, CALIFORNIA, TO EAST OF LAUGHLIN

Crossing my first state line was incredibly exciting; a real milestone. Depending on where you cross, there is usually a sign to declare where you are. I felt jubilant as I ran towards a large sign at the side of the road saying: "Welcome to Nevada". I knew I still had many more state lines to go, but there was something special about crossing the first one, especially as it had taken five days to reach it. I paused with the film crew so we could record the moment, and I was greeted by two lovely American guys who were there on holiday and also taking photos. Another opportunity seized for some witness statements.

I would only be covering 21 miles (33.8 km) through Nevada so I tried to take in as much as I could before we stopped for the night close to the next state line. It was similar to the desert scenery I had just been running through in California. I was running on the same stretch of road, making navigation nice and easy, surrounded by dry, flat sandy land dotted with green bushes. Up ahead I could see the mountains of Arizona rising above the horizon.

It was still extremely hot with no shade, so the crew decided to keep meeting me every couple of miles to check on me and give me more water and ice cubes. I would stuff my headband with ice cubes – this time putting it on my head rather than wrapping it around my wrist. I must have looked ridiculous, but it was an excellent way to keep me cool. Becky ran with me for a couple of miles and then Paul joined me through Laughlin for my final five of the day, which made a huge difference and took my mind off the heat. As the sun set, we were treated to a spectacular sky with rays of pink, orange, red and purple light spreading out above us in a fan shape. Stopping for the end of the day near the state line for Arizona was a huge psychological boost. There were still hundreds of miles to go to New York, but I was two states down by the end of day five, and about to enter my third.

12–19 SEPTEMBER
STATE THREE: ARIZONA
DISTANCE COVERED: 439.38 MILES (707.11 KM)
EAST OF LAUGHLIN TO SOUTH OF TEEC NOS POS

The following morning, Becky and I headed off in good spirits despite the fact we hadn't been able to sleep well. The temperature had remained high overnight at over 28°C (82°F), making it incredibly hot in the RV, even with the air conditioning on. "I ended up sleeping on the floor in my underwear as it was just too hot!" Becky admitted. We were excited because it was the end of the first week, and within 5 minutes of running, we would be crossing the Colorado River into Arizona, the Grand Canyon State.

On entering Arizona, we were still in quite an arid desert area but now the landscape was also dotted with the most beautiful red rock formations. It immediately became clear why it is known as one of the mountain states, as we hit an uphill stretch for the next 15 miles (24 km). We started to notice lots of full water bottles randomly scattered along the road with notes attached to them.

"They must have known we were coming," Becky joked.

The crew later discovered from a local fireman who signed a witness statement that the bottles were put there by the locals (and regularly replaced) in case of emergency, such as if a car broke down and the occupants were stranded till help arrived. The water would be very much needed in this remote area due to the extreme heat.

There had been another milestone moment when we crossed the state line – but we had missed it! We had passed from the Pacific to the Mountain time zone, but our watches hadn't updated. Jenny felt awful that she hadn't realized but it was only an hour's time difference and it was an easy mistake to make. I wasn't concerned as I tried not to worry about situations that were out of my control. As long as I got in the miles I needed for the day, and I was able to get enough sleep, I didn't mind.

A perk of Arizona was the wide hard shoulders on the roads. I thought it meant I could relax a bit more, as I didn't have to watch out continually for the cars coming towards me, but I was proved wrong. A local sheriff we had met earlier had warned us they had been having trouble with drivers under the influence. Unfortunately, we encountered one such person in the middle of the day when a vehicle passed us and its curious driver pulled over to see what we were up to. Jenny took the opportunity to get them to sign a witness statement but alarmingly they could barely hold the pen, let alone drive, as they seemed to be incredibly drunk. They nearly reversed into the support vehicle as they drove off. "I'm calling 911 to let them know," Jenny said. It didn't feel right to just let them drive off knowing the state they were in. They could have easily caused a serious accident or even killed someone. This made me feel even more uneasy about running beside the road.

I didn't have much further to go before I would be off-road again, but this was both a blessing and a curse. Between Kingman and Flagstaff, the most direct route would have been along the straight interstate I-40. However, runners aren't allowed on it as it is too dangerous, plus it was forbidden by Guinness for the record attempt. I had no option but to wiggle my way round a variety of small roads and dirt tracks that weaved like a snake north and south of the highway, not just adding miles but also hills.

Despite this, my body was feeling remarkably strong, which was a massive bonus. At one point I ran through a field of cows being guarded by a very large bull who seemed determined to come over and investigate me more closely. He was huge and very intimidating! At this point, the support car was with me going along a dirt track through the field, so I ran with the car between him and me just in case he decided to charge – it was just as well I was running in kit in my favourite colour of pink and not red!

While the off-road route made running difficult, the scenery was incredible. There were snow-topped mountain peaks and lush green pine forests all around, so it was much more exhilarating than running beside a long, traffic-filled road. One section took us to a dried-up river bed that was impossible for the support car to drive along. We couldn't find an alternative route so it was decided I should do the next 5 miles (8 kilometres) or so alone, packed up with as much water and as many snacks as I could carry.

I loved being in the middle of nowhere, zigzagging across rivers, scrambling over boulders, and fighting my way through long grass, where I spotted wild pigs and an elk. It was all part of the adventure and took my mind off the mileage count as I had to focus on getting to the end of the day in one piece, and without getting lost in the wilderness. In particular, I had to stay alert for rattle snakes as we had been warned there were a lot around at this time of year. I was constantly concentrating on the ground in front of me to check I wasn't about to step on one. The crew had given me a Sharpie pen just in case I was bitten. I was told I should use it to circle the bite and write beside it the time I was bitten. I would then draw another loop later around the swollen area, again noting the time, so doctors could see the progression of my reaction to the poison and work out how much anti-venom to give. A good idea but it did make me laugh. If I was unfortunate enough to get bitten, I certainly wouldn't have remembered to write anything down as I would more likely be panicking!

While I was enjoying my off-road adventures in Arizona feeling like Indiana Jones, it was a tough stage for the crew whose experience was more like *Breaking Bad*. After getting a puncture, they then got lost when they went to seek help. After asking for directions, they wandered up an isolated dirt track that made them feel extremely uneasy. It appeared they had stumbled upon some sort of drug den with a crystal meth set-up. They scrambled to get away as quickly as possible before encountering any of the local hoodlums. Luckily they managed to get help with the puncture from a passing motorist, who warned them they were in a notoriously crime-ridden area, and shouldn't be there for long unarmed. It was a really dangerous and quite scary experience for them, and made us realize how vulnerable we were because much of the time we had no mobile phone signal. From then on, Jenny arranged to have a satellite phone with them at all times. Jan also bought pepper spray and a shovel the next time they stopped at a store and VW, our car sponsors, came up trumps by providing the vehicle with new tyres that they arranged to be put on the next day.

Running through Flagstaff I wasn't completely alone, as I was lucky to have a Facebook friend, Breanna Kay Cornel, who lives in the area, come out and run with me for a few miles on two consecutive days. She knows the area well, so she was an excellent guide and stopped me getting lost. It meant so much to me that she came out to join me and it was wonderful to get to know her and her lovely dog, Sophie, who she brought out on the second day. I was quite envious of how Sophie could spring and sprint up and down the mountain paths with such unbridled energy. She made it look so easy. She also made me miss my own dog, Rani.

Of course, I was missing the rest of my family at home too. I knew Tim, our three grown-up children and three grandchildren would be constantly keeping up to date with how I was doing via all my trackers and updates from the crew. I had given my grandchildren, Theo, then aged nine, Finley, nearly six, and Millie, three, a large map of America with my route marked on it so they could track my progress. My family knows that during events like this I rarely contact anyone – and avoid knowing about what is happening in the world in general – as I find it too much of a distraction. I have to be in my own little bubble so I can focus on the task in hand. Even if I had wanted to call them we rarely had a decent phone signal, but I was able to get a few messages from them via social media which was lovely. The crew would often read them out to me during my lunch breaks to give me a boost. I couldn't wait till Tim would be joining me so I could see him, and he could fill me in with all the news from home.

The following day, as I ran alone along a forest track, there were a lot of shooting sounds which was disconcerting – but I had been warned to expect it as it was hunting season. When Jenny and Jan didn't arrive at a pre-arranged spot on the route to meet me, I started to feel a slight panic that perhaps I was lost. I had no means of contacting the crew because I never ran with my mobile phone. I find it too distracting and it would have been something extra to carry when I already needed to use the pockets and pouches on my vest for snacks and water. Not only that, in this remote area I rarely had a signal to make carrying a mobile worth it, even the GPS trackers weren't working all the time because of the poor signal. It wasn't usually a problem because the crew knew my exact route and could find me along it, but on this occasion, I was worried I had gone off course. Through the trees, I saw a large 4x4 coming towards me, so I madly waved my arms to flag it down for help. When the driver pulled over and wound down the window I was momentarily taken aback to see the car full of hunters in face paint and full-on camouflage gear, holding crossbows. Despite their slightly scary appearance, they were very kind and friendly. They agreed to let me use one of their phones which luckily did have a signal. As I only knew Tim's mobile number by heart, I had to call him at home and then tell him to contact Jan and let her know where I was. The hunters kindly gave me a bottle of water and offered to give me a lift to take me to the crew but of course that wasn't allowed!

When the crew and I were finally reunited, it turned out I had been on the correct route but they missed our meet up because the support car had become stuck in the mud. They had to wedge logs and rocks behind the back wheels to free it. Jenny and Jan expressed concern about my appearance when they saw me.

"You look like you are losing too much weight," Jan said. "Have you been eating all your snacks?"

I realized I hadn't. It hadn't been intentional but thanks to running large sections without the crew there to remind and cajole me to eat, I had been forgetting because I hadn't felt hungry. Plus, I simply couldn't carry enough food on me to keep up the calorie intake I needed. I was burning more than 6,000 calories a day. I tried not to worry about it as we would soon be out of the off-road section so it would be easier for me to get regular snacks again via the support car.

After running nearly 440 miles (708 km) through Arizona, on top of the 280 miles (451 km) I had done through California and 21 miles (34 km) in Nevada, I was still feeling surprisingly strong. However, the off-road terrain was causing extra stress on my ankle joints, especially the left one, as they had to work harder to keep me stable. I have had a problem with this joint since 2008 when I twisted it badly in Chile's Atacama desert. I was competing in the 150-mile (241-km) Atacama Crossing at the time, a self-sufficiency staged race. I had managed to push through the pain to finish first female and 20th overall, but it had left me with some long-term weakness, which I worried had flared up again now.

On inspection, Fiona noticed I had a bruise going up the outside of my leg which could possibly mean I had a stress fracture. The normal treatment for this would be rest, but that wasn't an option for me when I was in the middle of a world record attempt. I couldn't even afford to have one day off. The clock started ticking on the world record time when I left City Hall in L.A. and would keep ticking until I reached City Hall in New York. If I took a rest day, it would be an extra day on the record which I didn't want. I wasn't just here to run across America, I wanted to do it in the fastest time possible, especially as I knew I was also running against Sandra.

Fiona taped my ankle up to give the joint some more support, and I just had to do my best to ignore it. I was aware of a dull ache but it wasn't getting worse and it didn't feel nearly as bad as it had in Atacama so I decided I wasn't going to worry about it. It was a relief when the off-road section came to an end and I was back to running along a wide hard shoulder on Route 89. However, there were some sections where the hard shoulder completely disappeared and the camber would make it feel worse again. I found it easier at these points to run down the centre of the road, so long as there was no traffic.

Running on the same road all day became very dull and the effects of the altitude were making me feel like I was always running uphill. I found listening to music (with a headphone in just one ear so I could still hear the traffic) helped to pass the time and distract me from how tired I felt. Listening to some of my favourite songs helps me focus on something different, and on occasions gets me singing as I run – thankfully there was rarely anyone around to hear me! One of my favourite songs is "Fly Me to the Moon". My family are sick of it as at home I sing it every morning as I'm going downstairs to make coffee, and I still only know the first verse!

Another way I passed the time was to set myself mini targets, such as to keep running at a certain pace until I reached the crew at our next pre-arranged meeting spot. I also kept my mind occupied by just thinking. Running is my time to ponder anything and everything, whatever pops into my head. At other times, I just tried to stay in the moment and take in as much of my surroundings as I could, as well as being alert for passing traffic. There wasn't much to see around me or many vehicles on this particular stretch of road but the sky above me was beautiful. It became filled with different shades of pink, red and orange as the sunset curved above me. I felt as though it was wrapping me up in a big hug.

Another issue I noticed when I finished for the day was that my feet were starting to get swollen and puffy. I knew this could happen so I had packed extra pairs of trainers half a size and a full size up to what I usually wore. It wasn't just me; the crew were also finding their feet were swollen and larger than usual. It must have been down to the heat as well as the altitude we were now at.

I had been alternating wearing three different types of Hoka trainers, to save wearing one pair out and to mix things up to keep my feet comfortable. We realized that if I carried on needing larger sizes, I wouldn't have enough pairs to alternate them. Jenny told me not to worry, she would contact Tim and see if he could bring some extra pairs when he joined us. I was lucky to have Hoka as one of my sponsors, so they were happy to supply me with whatever I needed, for which I was very grateful. Tim was also tasked with bringing out Yorkshire tea bags, Marmite and vegetable stock cubes as the crew hadn't been able to find any of these in the US and were missing a good old British brew!

Apart from my sore ankle, I had made it through the first of the mountain states relatively unscathed despite all the potential dangers. I hoped my luck would continue into the next one. The wonderfully named Teec Nos Pos was my last stop in Arizona before I crossed into my fourth state.

19–22 SEPTEMBER
STATE FOUR: NEW MEXICO
DISTANCE COVERED: 171.32 MILES (275.71 KM)
SOUTH OF TEEC NOS POS TO NORTH OF CHAMA

"Welcome to New Mexico, the Land of Enchantment" read the sign, which would have been easy to miss as I crossed the state line as it wasn't very obvious on the side of the road. My time here would be far from magical as I would be spending the vast majority running along Route 64. I knew from driving this stretch that it was going to be incredibly monotonous running beside the same long, straight, very hilly road day after day, with just trees to look at. An added issue was there was no hard shoulder along most of the road, so I would always have to be alert for traffic and dive off the road if need be.

I was now two weeks into the world record attempt, and with little to distract me along Route 64, I did start to wonder how Sandra was getting on with her run. So far, I had tried to resist asking the crew for updates on how she was doing. I knew they would never tell me unless I asked. Sometimes when I did they challenged me: "Do you really want to know?" And most of the time I didn't. I was curious to know how many miles she was doing each day, but I also knew that information would make me compare myself to her and feel additional pressure.

But at the end of my first day running through New Mexico, I succumbed to temptation and just had to find out. It was a rare evening when we had a strong mobile phone signal so after checking my messages from family and friends while having a massage, I logged on to Facebook to see Sandra's posts. She was making good progress averaging 57 miles (92 km) a day, passing through Yosemite National Park and the Inyo National Forest on her route through California. In all of her pictures, she looked strong, happy and glowing. It made my heart sink. I knew I shouldn't have been comparing myself to her, particularly as I had been on the road for a few days more than she had, but I couldn't help it.

Seeing how easy she was making everything look made me feel totally inadequate. Not only was I now feeling tired and drawn, I was starting to get a constant pain at the back of my right leg, particularly behind the knee. Fiona kept asking me if my knee was sore as she was well aware of the surgery I had the year before, but I always replied, "no" as I wasn't experiencing pain in the actual knee joint, just everywhere around it. Even just turning over in bed at night was making it hurt.

I bet Sandra isn't feeling this way, I thought. *Am I really up to this?*

After tormenting myself for too long, I realized it was time to put the phone down, and not look at Sandra's posts again. "Comparison is the thief of joy" is a well-known expression, and in this case, it was also stealing my confidence and faith in my own ability. I had to forget about Sandra, focus on myself and stick to my plan. I banished my concerns about the pain in my leg. I had to accept that some level of pain from all the running I was doing was now par for the course. I knew what I had to do – keep going, and keep taking one day at a time. Get to my bed, get up, get running, get to the first stage, get to the second stage, get to my bed again. Each day I did this was another day closer to New York.

Day 14 was another hot day with lots of elevation, especially in the second half of the day when we climbed up to 6,000 feet (1,829 m). Running in the heat of the day was tough but the crew were looking after me well. When I reached the milestone of 800 miles (1,287 km), they bought me an Oreo sandwich ice cream to celebrate – my favourite and it had never tasted so good. Not long after, two lovely Native Americans stopped at the support vehicle after seeing me run past and offered to be witnesses. They also said they would perform a wind and rain dance to encourage the weather to cool down for me. Sadly it didn't seem to work but it's the thought that counts!

As I had spent nearly all of my time in New Mexico running along Route 64, I started to wonder if this was the longest road in America. This got us all thinking and the crew later looked it up. We discovered that the longest road is in fact Route 20, stretching from Boston, Massachusetts to Newport, Oregon. A total of 12 states, and 3,365 miles (5,415 km)!

Towards the end of the following day I ran through Dulce where lots of people came out to cheer me on as I ran past. My day was brightened up thanks to a group of girls and a young man joining me for the last 2 miles. They were members of the Jicarilla Apache Nation, who had met my film crew earlier in the day. They told Carol and Susie that their tribal history involved a huge running race. Running was very much part of their tradition and ancestry, so they were very excited about coming out to run with me.

Those who have met me know I love to chat, but on this challenge I found talking was taking up too much energy, particularly by the end of the day. So while I didn't have much I was able to say to them, I loved hearing about their nation's history, their lives and their interest in running. One of the women later sent a message to thank me. She said the run with me was the longest distance she had run since leaving school several years ago. She wrote: "I really enjoyed running with you. You've inspired me to get back into it and try to run for longer next time." This really lifted my spirits after a tiring day as this is what I wanted my run to be all about – inspiring others to take on a challenge of their own.

We had been shocked when a white oil worker had told us "never to trust the Native Americans" as we ran through their reservation in Dulce. Of course, we ignored his prejudiced warning. Every Native American we met was exceedingly warm and friendly. One in particular went out of his way to accommodate us on an overnight stop. While I was running my final miles of the day, Paul had arranged to park the RV up for the night on the forecourt of a shopping outlet. He and Becky had started preparing my evening meal when a lone Native American approached and said we could stay the night at his place down the road. He offered to let us use his shower to freshen up, do our laundry in his washing machine, and said he would be able to supply fresh water to replenish our tanks. Paul and Becky were amazed by his generous offer. They jumped at the chance to have a hot shower outside the RV and knew everyone else would feel the same. The Native American introduced himself as Francisco, and he said he was an Apache.

"You are the first Apache I have ever met," Paul told him.

"You are the first Englishman I have ever met!" he replied.

Francisco had been born and educated on the reservation before leaving to go to college. He then returned to work there after qualifying as an accountant. He's since retired and now breeds horses on a ranch near his home with more than 500 animals.

I was delighted to reach the RV at Francisco's home to be told we could park there for the night. I couldn't thank him enough for his hospitality as he invited us to use his shower. As I wanted to get to bed as quickly as possible, I stuck to my usual routine of showering in the RV but the male crew members were grateful to be able to use Francisco's bathroom, while the women showered in his mother's house next door. He even provided fresh towels for everyone. Paul said it was a privilege to see inside Francisco's home, where his walls were adorned with pictures of his family, stretching back to his great-grandparents in their native dress, alongside Native American artefacts.

We ate supper as usual in the RV and Francisco kindly brought us some chicken wings he'd cooked. After thanking him again, I retired early for the evening to get as much rest as I could, while the crew stayed up a little longer having a wonderful time listening to Francisco's fascinating stories. He promised to make them an authentic Apache breakfast of bacon and beans in the morning and said he could arrange for the village Medicine Man to come and give us a traditional Apache blessing at sunrise. Unfortunately, as I would have to start running before the sun came up, I wouldn't be able to stay for this, but Paul and Jan said they would, and then catch up with me in the RV by lunchtime as usual.

I was woken up several times in the night by the sound of coyotes barking in the distance. Francisco's dogs were doing an excellent job of keeping them away from his property by barking back loudly, but this did make it difficult to sleep. I managed to get a bit of shut-eye before setting off just before 5 a.m. with Becky by my side, shortly followed by Jenny and Fiona in the support car. I felt sad that I would miss the Apache blessing but I had no choice: the record had to remain my priority and, for that, we had to stick to our usual schedule. Paul and Jan excitedly told us all about it later.

The Medicine Man had arrived just before sunrise. Paul said he had been hoping he would be in Native American dress with a headdress full of feathers but instead he was in the modern attire of jeans, a sky-blue hoodie and paint-splattered brown shoes. The pair were told that for the blessing to be given, they would have to give the Medicine Man a gift of something that was unique to them. Jan sacrificed some of her precious and valuable Yorkshire teabags, while Paul gave him a signed copy of my first book, *Beyond Impossible* (I hope he later enjoyed reading it!). Paul then had to roll a cigarette and hand it to the Medicine Man. Being a non-smoker, he didn't do this very elegantly, but it was good enough to pass inspection by the Medicine Man, and the blessing began. Jan and Paul stood outside shoulder to shoulder, facing the sunrise, while the Medicine Man stood facing them with his back to the sun. He took the cigarette and lit it, accepted their gifts, and then spoke in Apache tongue, chanting for a while and pausing to spit on the ground. He then took a lighter and lit some corn kernels that he produced from his pocket, all beautifully timed with the sun rising over the mountains on the horizon behind him.

"The whole blessing lasted for what seemed like ten minutes and it was so moving and deeply meaningful, especially when choreographed with the rising sun. I was filled with emotion," Paul told us later as he vividly recalled the experience. "I was moved to tears despite not understanding a word of what had actually been said!"

Jan agreed: "It was such a privilege and something I will never forget."

Afterwards the Medicine Man told them he had asked the Sun God for a safe onward journey for us all, and in particular, for me. The pair enjoyed breakfast with Francisco before saying goodbye to our new friend. We were all overwhelmed by his kindness and generosity, inviting six complete strangers into his home. He had shown us all nothing but respect and had been the perfect host.

While I was disappointed that I had missed the blessing, the final day in New Mexico was one of excitement for me. I knew this was the day my husband, Tim, was flying out to Denver, Colorado, along with Sophie. I couldn't wait to see Tim again and to meet Sophie in person at last. There was a time when I had kept Tim away from my running challenges. It is hard to explain but I felt I had to keep my sport and my home life separate, as running had given me back some of my identity that I had somehow lost when I got married and had children. I liked the fact that when I was competing I was Mimi, an ultrarunner. Not "Mrs Anderson" or "Emma/Ruaraidh/Harri's mum" (as much as I also loved having these roles).

Tim was keen to see more of this crazy running world that had so captivated his wife. I wasn't a runner when we first met and he was bemused and baffled when I went from being a stay-at-home mother to our three children to an ultrarunning devotee. I used to dislike running and loved my home comforts but then voluntarily started hitting the trails for hours on end and taking on races that involved camping in the middle of nowhere. He asked to join the crew when I ran JOGLE but initially I wasn't sure if it was a good idea. As he wasn't a runner himself, I assumed he wouldn't understand what it would take to be an indispensable crew member. I also worried that as he was my husband, he wouldn't be able to be objective when he saw me in pain. Would he try to stop me carrying on at times when I was struggling, when what I actually needed was encouragement?

When he refused to take no for an answer and joined the crew for JOGLE halfway through the record attempt, I learnt my assumptions couldn't have been more wrong. I discovered he was the best crew member I could have wished for. He knows me so well, he knows when I need encouragement to go on when I think I have nothing left, when to say nothing, and when I need a hug. He will always be honest with me so can tell me if I need to stop for my own good if I try to push too far through the pain. I wouldn't have achieved the JOGLE world record, or many of the things I have done since, without him by my side. His love has given me the strength to believe in myself and enable me to follow my dreams. I knew having him join the crew now was going to make a huge difference as my journey across America was only going to get tougher the longer it went on.

CHAPTER THREE

SO FAR, SO GOOD

22–27 SEPTEMBER
STATE FIVE: COLORADO
DISTANCE COVERED: 304.63 MILES (490.25 KM)
NORTH OF CHAMA TO EAST OF HOLLY

Thinking about seeing Tim put a spring in my step, which was very much needed once I passed into Colorado. The hills were relentless, with the elevation going over 10,000 feet (3,048 m). Running at altitude is harder work because there is less oxygen in the air. The crew were feeling the effects going about their usual activities too, and they were quickly becoming breathless. Preparing meals was also more of a challenge for them, as they discovered food cooks differently at altitude due to the difference in atmospheric pressure compared to when at sea level. Foods that required boiling, such as pasta, took much longer to cook. There was no respite for me as the downhill sections were as steep as the uphill ones, putting an extra strain on my quads. I tried to stay focused on ticking the miles off, as each one was taking me closer to Tim.

I had entered Colorado on the sixteenth day of my run just after lunch, where I was greeted with massive cheers and whoops of celebration from a couple who were on holiday taking photos by the state sign. "Welcome to colourful Colorado," they said, echoing the message written on it. Colorado certainly was colourful. I know America is famous for its beautiful "fall" but this was the first time since starting in California that I actually noticed the change of season in all its glory. I was surrounded by autumn colours as I ran, with the leaves on the trees changing from vibrant greens to bright yellows, deep reds and golden browns, all against a backdrop of mountains. It was spectacular. Sometimes the colour was so dazzling it didn't seem real. It felt as though I was running through an impressionist painting.

But while the leaves were gradually starting to change, the weather went from summer to autumn in an instant. As I ran up the mountain road, one minute it was a sunny and hot 25°C (77°F), the next the wind picked up, replacing the sunshine with heavy rain and hail that battered me. I was struggling to control my body temperature as I had been sweating heavily when the weather had been warm, and now that sweat was going to bring my body temperature down too much. Although I didn't want to waste time having an unscheduled stop, I knew from my previous experience racing in sub-zero temperatures that I would need to get more layers on fast to prevent hypothermia setting in.

In ultramarathons I had run in places such as the Arctic, it had often been hypothermia, not lack of endurance, that had forced many people to drop out. Jenny and Fiona, who were in the support vehicle that afternoon, had left me about 15 minutes earlier, which meant I had to keep running. Thankfully the film crew drove past and came to the rescue, lending me some jogging bottoms and an extra top. The dry clothes made all the difference, enabling me to continue the long climb on the day's route, up to over 10,000 feet (3,048 m), feeling much better. I passed an interesting sign along the Continental Divide which informed me I was at the "Great Divide", where rainfall drains on one side into the Pacific Ocean and on the other side into the Atlantic.

The relentless rain and the uphill climb made for a testing day. There were numerous hairpin turns and it was often hard to see cars approaching round the tight bends, especially as the mountainside was also dense with trees. Fiona had to keep driving ahead of me, stopping at the corners to alert oncoming vehicles of my presence. For the last 3 hours towards the end of the day the thunderstorm continued, with lightning flashing across the sky, followed seconds later by a loud clap of thunder rumbling angrily overhead. It was twilight as I came off the mountain and the combination of the light and the rain created a natural phenomenon I have never seen anything like before. In front of me there were two pillars of a rainbow on my path. It was a stunning sight to behold and a beautiful end to what had been a long and tiring day.

I was delighted when I finally reached the RV for the night, especially as a few moments after my arrival, Jenny pulled up in the other support car having picked up Tim and Sophie. They had to take several bus journeys after their flight to reach a point where Jenny could collect them and had been amazed by the stormy skies I was running under, as well as delighting in seeing the beautiful rainbows.

I was ecstatic to see Tim, but our reunion wasn't passionate because kissing him was extremely painful! The sun and wind had left my lips chapped and swollen, and he decided since I had been away to grow a full-on beard – not a good combination! It was wonderful though to have a hug from him. You don't realize how much you'll miss someone until you are apart for a length of time. I had missed him more than I ever thought I would. He had been following my progress since day one and said he was impressed with how it was going and how positive I still was.

"You are well on track for the record!" he beamed.

He was also impressed with the slick crew operation that was taking place, as he saw how the team could operate in the tiny RV kitchen to cook up a feast and then tidy up without getting in each other's way. An arm would go between someone's legs to take a glass from a cupboard, a head would duck down in anticipation of another arm reaching for the top of a shelf. "It's like watching a ballet," Tim said.

I was also delighted to finally meet Sophie. While we had talked lots over the phone before the challenge, I hadn't actually met her in person yet. We instantly hit it off and I knew I had made the right decision asking her to be part of the team.

"Welcome aboard!" I told her. "Thank you so much for coming out to support me."

"It's great to be here," Sophie replied. "This is a dream come true for me. I love going on adventures!"

As the rest of us had spent so long in one another's company, it was wonderful to have a new vibe with Tim and Sophie among us. They were feeling fresh and raring to go, with Sophie already bursting with excitement about exploring a new continent and culture, and she was particularly impressed by the range of snacks available in America.

"The scenery on the journey here was amazing," she told us, as they had taken a long bus ride to reach us at the foot of the Rockies. "And can you believe I found coffee nut flavour M&Ms at the airport? They're delicious!"

While I was overjoyed to see Tim and Sophie, their arrival was also tinged with sadness as it meant the following evening I would have to say goodbye to Becky and Paul. The next morning Becky and I ran together for the last time, a very special occasion and one that I will never forget. Once she stopped running with me to start her packing, I carried on towards Alamosa. Although the road I was on was flat, we were still at 7,500 ft (2,286 m) of altitude.

After a quick lunch and leaving for my second stint of the day, a Facebook friend of mine called Jeff Owsley drove up to see me. As well as signing a witness statement and running with me, he had also arranged a welcome committee in Alamosa. Unfortunately, it had taken me slightly longer than I had anticipated to reach the town so many people had dispersed by the time I got there, but it was lovely to see a large group of patient people including children holding up signs saying: "Congratulations – you have just run a third of the way across the USA!" There were high fives and hugs all round. Jeff carried on running with me through the town and told me Alamosa is known as the Gateway to Great Sand Dunes National Park. The most famous feature of this National Park is an enormous dune field, which contains the tallest sand dunes in North America. I would have loved to have seen them but there was, of course, no time to stop and pay them a visit. I was also relieved I wouldn't be running over them, as I know from my previous desert ultras how energy sapping running up and over sand dunes can be.

After a final dinner together in the RV, it was time for me to say a sad farewell to Becky and Paul. They had been such brilliant support and company and we celebrated the fact they had helped me get a third of the way across America. I couldn't imagine what it was going to be like to continue without them. Becky just "got" me. Sometimes it was as though she could read my mind. For example, on one particular day with only about an hour to go until I finished, the temperature had fallen and I thought how nice it would be to have a hot water bottle in my bed when I got into it that evening. I had brought one with me from the UK as I know when I am tired I often feel the cold more, especially at night. When I finally arrived back at the RV having finished my running for the day, I asked Becky if she could do this, only for her to tell me she already had!

Paul had also been wonderful at driving and parking the RV – not an easy thing to do. Tim would now be taking over this role and he had been given lots of instructions from Paul on how everything worked, alongside a full tour in and outside the massive vehicle to find out where everything was. There was a lot to take in, not just on how to drive and park it but also how to refuel, sort out the water and waste tanks and connect all the electrics when needed.

"Thanks for your support and encouragement. I'm going to miss you. You have done such an amazing job," I told them both as we said our goodbyes.

"Keep going. We know you can do it. Just keep taking one day at a time," Becky advised me. Knowing the full history of my eating disorder and relationship with food, she then added: "I'm so proud of how much you are eating. You are doing everything right. Just make sure you keep eating the food you're given."

Members of the crew had given me a telling off on more than one occasion for not eating enough. One evening, I had chucked away half of the wrap I had been handed on the run (hoping nobody had seen my silent revolt) as I knew I didn't have many more miles to go that day and I would be eating again when I arrived at the RV. Becky had been on to me and berated me for it later. I knew she was right as it was vital to eat what I was given but I found it all too easy to revert to my bad habits if allowed, as I still didn't have much of an appetite when running. I knew I would have to keep Becky's words in mind when I was feeling rebellious over my eating plan. After she left, I only threw a small amount of my food away a couple of times over the course of the run.

The following morning, it was on with the show, and the wet weather continued which made running less enjoyable. There were several times when we had to change course, as flooding had made our intended route impassable. I wasn't too happy about this as the side roads were often laid with gravel which I was finding uncomfortable to run on; it made my legs and core work harder to stabilize my balance. The main roads weren't much more pleasant, as I had to endure spray from the cars and lorries again when they drove past me. It was slightly terrifying as even though I was wearing my usual high vis and had lights on, I knew the conditions and surface spray would make it harder for the drivers to see me, especially as they wouldn't have been expecting to see a runner on these types of roads. I had to be on my guard at all times, watching the cars as they drove towards me and jumping off the road if I felt a vehicle was not going to give me enough room as they passed. My fear was compounded by the fact I had been hit by a car during my JOGLE world record. I was struck by the wing mirror so forcibly that it snapped off the vehicle, leaving me with an injured, but thankfully not broken, arm. I really hoped history wouldn't repeat itself. I also knew of numerous ultrarunners and cyclists who had been badly injured after being hit by cars when travelling across America.

Something else that I had experienced when running the length of Great Britain had recurred, and it was making it very difficult for me to run. Over the past few days, I had been having issues with my bladder, making going to the loo extremely painful. I knew there was nothing for it but to ease back on the running; otherwise it would only get worse. I decided that in the afternoon I would power walk for the rest of the day to give my bladder time to recover. I worried about how this would affect my pace, but by this stage it wasn't that much slower than the running I was able to do.

My pace was something I often fretted about. I knew that people would be following my run via Strava and it made me worry about what they would think about my progress, and criticize me for being too slow. I had to keep reminding myself that covering the target distance by the end of each day was what mattered. Despite my aching bladder I managed to reach 58 miles (93 km) that day and I also hit 1,000 miles (1,609 km) in total – the crew played the Proclaimers song "500 Miles" as I arrived at the support vehicle to celebrate. They also cheered me up by telling me they had passed the time waiting for me to reach them by doing 50 squats. They certainly got a few funny looks from passing cars!

The power walking that day had been the right call, as it made a huge difference to my bladder as well as lifting my mood. Walking also gave me the opportunity to take in more of my surroundings. One stretch of road was an arachnophobe's nightmare. The Tarmac was constantly covered in scuttling tarantulas. I'm not scared of spiders, but their size and movement did send a slight shiver down my spine. I tried to pass them as quickly as possible without treading on any. We learned later that these were the males on their annual migration to find females to mate with. When they reach about eight years old, they gang up in groups and set out, using their senses of touch and vibration to locate the females. At this particular spot, they had to cross a busy road to reach them, meaning many of them sadly got squashed by cars.

A much more pleasant encounter with the natural world came when I was back running along Route 160, heading towards Walsenburg. There was a wide hard shoulder to run on so I felt a bit more relaxed and could enjoy the scenery.

The rain had finally relented and the sun was starting to break through the clouds when suddenly I noticed hundreds of butterflies starting to fly past me. The change in weather must have provided the ideal conditions for them to hatch. For about 3 miles (5 kilometres), these green and yellow winged beauties fluttered by, beating their wings on the warm air. If I stretched out my arms they would land on me. It was magical, another treat from colourful Colorado.

So far, there had been very few mornings when I had woken up and thought: *I don't want to get up and go running today*. But on 25 September, I thought exactly that. My sore bladder and resulting drop in pace from having to power walk had made me feel despondent. It would have been so easy to tell the crew when our alarms went off at 4.30 a.m.: "Let's start half an hour later today and have a lie in." But I knew I couldn't do that. It would have thrown our usual routine out of sync and it was important we all kept to the same timings as we were working as a team. It would also waste precious time when I was up against the clock to gain the world record. An hour extra in bed now would mean an extra hour on the record time. I had to act as if I was getting up and going to work. There are lots of times when you don't want to get up and go, but you have to get on with it when it's your job. My job right now was trying to break a world record.

Perhaps I should have stayed in bed though – that afternoon, everything seemed to go wrong! I got stung by ants when I stopped for an al fresco pee, my hamstring was sore which was slowing me down and I had to stop to change my clothes to be more comfortable. All very frustrating as it took up precious time. Then Tim had a mishap with the RV which would prove expensive to repair.

Paul had taken Tim through a checklist of everything the driver needed to do before leaving after an overnight stop. This included walking around the RV and ensuring each storage unit was closed, unplugging the electric and water supply, and removing the chocks from under the wheels and the steps to the door (the latter is something Tim had forgotten to do when driving the camper van during my JOGLE world record, so we lost those steps somewhere in Wales!).

One of the clever gadgets that the RV possessed was an awning that electronically unrolled and refolded from the side of the vehicle at the press of a button. When in use it provided some extra space for us outside the RV with shelter from the sun and rain. Obviously, this needed to be retracted before driving off, but on this occasion as Tim set off in the dark early in the morning, he forgot! As he rushed to reach our pre-arranged lunch stop before I did – having to factor in time to stop and clean and refuel the RV – he was alarmed to hear a loud crunching noise as he sped along a deserted main road. This was the sound of the awning tearing off its mountings and parting company with the RV. It was still dark when he surveyed the damage so he could see there was some twisted metal sticking out from the side of the RV but it didn't look dangerous. He carried on his way, desperate not to leave me in limbo waiting for him and my lunch.

As it was becoming light he overtook me and Jenny. We immediately saw what had happened and flew into a panic, waving frantically to get Tim to stop. The metal bars were actually sticking out at 90 degrees to the side of the RV, a definite danger of striking something like a telegraph pole on the side of the road. Thankfully Tim saw us and stopped, along with some police officers who were passing at the time. They managed to bend the bars back and stick them down with plastic ties and tape so they were no longer a hazard. I couldn't believe Tim had done this, but I couldn't be mad as I had to stay focused on running. We would have to worry about the cost later. I knew he had a lot to remember with the RV too, especially as each morning he was under pressure to get it ready to go and then get to my lunch stop before I did so my food could be prepared on board. We did miss having the awning for the rest of the trip, but we were able to laugh about it.

On the plus side that day, when I ran through a Walmart car park a lovely lady called Chris saw me as she was about to leave with her shopping. She got out of her car to ask if I was the woman she had heard so much about running across America. She was also a fellow runner but had never tried to run ultra distances so she said she was in awe of what I was trying to achieve. I really enjoyed taking a few moments to chat to her. Meeting new people who were enthusiastic and inspired by my run always gave me a boost.

In the last section of Colorado, we said goodbye to Fiona and hello to her replacement physio, Beccy. Fiona had been a wonderful asset with her physio treatment and I couldn't thank her enough as we said our farewells. With her help, I had run more than 1,000 miles (1,609 km) in less than 18 days on the road. When she set off to the airport with Jenny the following morning, they drove past me waving goodbye when I realized I needed one more treatment from her. I was having a slight issue with my right leg and thankfully the rest of the support crew managed to flag them down further up the road so she could give me a quick massage before continuing her journey home.

After dropping Fiona off for her flight, Jenny then had to wait at the airport to collect Beccy so we were two crew members down, and I didn't have a physio available for the remainder of the day. Luckily, Fiona had taught Susie from the film crew how to do a basic calf massage, so she was able to help me out in the evening when my limbs were really starting to ache. She was terrified she would do it wrong, telling me: "I don't want to be the one responsible for messing up your knee or world record attempt!" But she did a fine job.

It was lovely to have the chance to spend some extra time chatting to her too. There weren't many opportunities we could do this since I always running or resting, while she was filming with Carol and then editing their footage every evening in their RV. We bonded over our shared love of Jack Russell terriers. I was amazed when Susie told me she had handed in her notice with a former employer in order to work for Carol and join us on the trip across America.

"When else would I ever get the opportunity to witness someone trying run from L.A. to New York?" she told me. "It is one of the best decisions I have ever made. I had no idea what to expect. I must admit I hadn't heard of ultrarunning before, but it sounded like a fun adventure, which is something I was definitely craving, and it hasn't disappointed."

Beccy arrived to find a runner whose mind was more than willing to keep ticking off the miles but whose body was less able. The bruising around my left ankle and shins had now disappeared but the whole of my right leg was constantly sore. My hamstring was particularly painful but Beccy was a whizz with the tape which allowed me to continue without it bothering me too much. It helped that I knew we were about to cross into my sixth state – Kansas. Although I was sad to say goodbye to Colorado, I was looking forward to running through Kansas as I knew it would be much flatter.

"Another state closer to New York," I whooped with joy as we crossed the state line.

27 SEPTEMBER–5 OCTOBER
STATE SIX: KANSAS
DISTANCE COVERED: 429.78 MILES (691.66 KM)
EAST OF HOLLY TO DREXEL

My joy at being in Kansas was short-lived. Although it is known as the Sunflower State, I found it far from bright and cheery. The scenery was very different compared to Colorado. Instead of being surrounded by beautiful mountains, I constantly ran past large fields full of corn that always looked as though it had been left for too long as it was so brown in colour. I found out this corn was destined to be food for the cows who live on giant cattle farms in the state. Red meat is big business in America and demand is high. We saw some of these farms where the cows are corralled into circular pens. The ground of the pens was covered in mud and the animals didn't seem to have much space. It was such a contrast to the way I was used to seeing cows in the UK, roaming free in a grassy green field. It was almost enough to turn me into a vegetarian. The smell of manure from these farms was also revolting. On the plus side, I heard a lot of birds singing sweetly and crickets chirping as I ran past the corn. On one evening just before the sun began to set, I saw the most spectacular sight, a murmuration of starlings. Their formations were breathtaking as they swooped and curled as one; I allowed myself a couple of minutes to pause and enjoy the spectacle.

When entering Kansas, we passed from the Mountain into the Central time zone, which meant another hour of lost sleep, and an extra hour of running in the dark each morning. We weren't quite sure where the time zone started but, having missed the last one, we decided that we would get up an hour early anyway. As it turned out, the time change didn't happen until a place called Kendall, 26 miles (42 km) further on.

Thankfully the mornings were now brightened up for me by Sophie's company. She really filled the void left by Becky. I had the occasional whinge to her about my aches and pains but she was very good at taking my mind off it and giving everything a positive slant. When I got cross and frustrated with myself for how few miles I had been able to cover in an hour because I was going so slowly, Sophie simply told me to forget the last hour and start again with the next one – perfect sense and it worked.

I loved hearing about her life and her running adventures. We laughed so much my face ached. She had left her job in 2016 to run across Scandinavia in 103 days. If anyone could understand her desire and drive to do that it was me. I also loved hearing how Sophie was finding it being a member of my crew. By now, they were all becoming exhausted. Their day was always longer than mine as once I went to bed, they would stay up to have a crew meeting to discuss the logistics for the following day. As well as planning the route, stops and meals, they would organize all the laundry, doing trips to laundrettes they could find along the way with one of the support cars. The washing up was another big job as there was a constant stream of it, all to be done in the tiny RV sink. Sophie and Tim had created a system for this in the evening which they were rather proud of. Tim said the pair of them would do the washing up, drying up and putting away "with such synchronization that Olympic synchronized swimmers would have been impressed."

I was so immensely grateful for their efforts. As the runner in the team, my job was to do the mileage each day. I literally didn't have to lift a finger to do anything else thanks to my amazing crew. All this was done on the back of very little sleep. The sleep deprivation combined with living in close quarters must have meant there were times when tempers inevitably frayed between them. Tim admitted he was unnecessarily short with Darren on one occasion shortly after he had just joined us. Darren arrived on 2 October to take over from Tim, who would soon be heading home (much to my sadness). New to our routine, Darren inadvertently upset Tim's aforementioned smooth washing up operation. In an effort to be helpful, he had put a dirty mug on the sideboard – but in the wrong place! Nothing you would normally get uptight about but for Tim running his tight ship at the time, it was a big deal, as it was upsetting his well-oiled machine. He was embarrassed to admit he told Darren off. To his credit, Darren took it on the chin and said no more – although I suspect he must have felt worried he was now going to be living with a strange obsessive crew member who spent a lot of time by the sink! I'm sure members of the crew bit their tongues a few times if I was a bit short with them when tired and frustrated. In situations like this it is impossible for everyone to get on all the time but, if there were any falling outs or resentments, they kept them all quiet from me.

I could tell Sophie was always tired in the mornings as she admitted she wasn't usually an early riser, but she was always upbeat about it.

"The one thing I'm not struggling with is sleeping," she told me one morning when I asked how she was coping. "I have discovered I can sleep at any time of day, anywhere! I have become the master of power naps!"

Jenny was very good at planning the schedule so the crew could have regular naps when needed, otherwise it would have been too dangerous for them to drive. Sophie was loving learning about the American way of life during our time on the road and was continuing to marvel at the variety of snacks they had on offer.

"Tim and I found eight different varieties of Snickers in a petrol station yesterday afternoon!" she told me. "We've vowed to try every one."

I'm sure they were capable of it. While the crew weren't joining me for many miles running, they were running around after me, so they were all building up big appetites as a result.

"Going to McDonalds with Tim was quite an experience," Sophie also recalled. "Has he ever been to one before? When he ordered a McFlurry, he asked for a McFluffy!"

This made me laugh out loud. Tim certainly would have been out of place in a McDonalds as it's not somewhere we ever usually went to eat, even when our kids were younger.

"The people we have been meeting are great too," Sophie went on. "They think what you are doing is fantastic but crazy. But do you know, most Americans don't want to talk to me about you, they just ask me if I knew Princess Diana!"

As we ran, we were treated to some of the most spectacular sunrises I have ever seen. Carol commented that at times it looked as though the sky was on fire. I rarely saw the sunset as it was always behind me and even when the crew told me how beautiful it was and I should turn and look, I often didn't have the energy to do so as I had to stay focused on moving forwards. If I stopped to look, I might not get going again. In the mornings I could take in the scenery more and enjoy a few chats, but by the afternoons I was digging deep and just thinking about getting the miles under my belt.

The inside of my nose was becoming very sore. I almost became obsessed with it, constantly picking at a scab that had formed within one of my nostrils, causing it to bleed and making it become even more painful. Perhaps subconsciously this was another way I was trying to take my mind off the distances I was running. Unfortunately, it probably made me look as though I was picking my nose all the time which must have been very unpleasant to see!

As the miles took their toll, little things really started to annoy me, and poor Carol felt the brunt of this when she was running behind me filming one afternoon. We were going along a monotonous road with the same horizontal landscape all around. The long, straight path ahead stretched all the way to the horizon miles away. As there was little change of scenery, it felt as though I wasn't making any progress and I was stuck in some kind of time loop where I was running the same stretch of road over and over.

I was tired and not my usual chirpy self as I was just trying to focus on getting each mile in the bank so I could finish for the day. But I was distracted from my thoughts because all I could hear behind me was an annoying "squeak, squeak, squeak". Glancing behind me I could see it was Carol jogging along holding her camera and the irritating noise was coming from her trainers. They squeaked every time her foot landed. I tried to see the funny side and block it out, but it really started to get to me, and I knew I couldn't carry on for another mile with the distracting accompaniment. Eventually I snapped.

"Will you please stop running quite so close as all I can hear are those annoying squeaky trainers!" I told her, trying to be as polite as I could. "Perhaps you could run slightly further back so I can't hear the squeaking quite as much?"

"I'm so sorry!" she said and immediately stopped following me.

The relief at having peace and quiet again as I continued was immense! I did feel guilty though for getting cross with Carol so I apologized to her at the end of the day. Luckily, she thought it was hilarious.

"All this time I have been worried it was my heavy breathing, puffing and huffing behind you trying to keep up while carrying my camera that would be annoying!" she laughed.

On most days Carol ran behind me at some stage for a short time to film me. At other times, she would be waiting for me as I approached, with her camera set up by the side of the road on a tripod. I never knew when she might pop up. She promised to buy some new trainers at the next shop we passed so she wouldn't be so distracting again.

After the altitude of Colorado I had been looking forward to some easier running, because Kansas is supposed to be flat. I didn't find this to be the case though as our route was quite undulating, which I felt keenly, especially now I was getting fatigued and my hamstring was quite sore. If it got too bad, I had to resort to power walking because even the tiniest uphill felt like a mountain climb. I was still finding running on the same road slightly demoralizing too. My legs felt as though they were full of lead.

At times, the road had no hard shoulder and I found it difficult keeping an eye on the traffic coming towards me, wondering whether they would go around me or come straight at me. On several occasions – more than I care to remember – it seemed as though they would make a bee-line for me which was pretty terrifying, especially as there really wasn't anywhere for me to go. It was made even worse in Kansas by particularly strong winds. Unfortunately, our time passing through coincided with an unseasonable bout of very windy weather. Battling the headwinds was a nightmare as it made my progress feel much slower. When heavy trucks drove past, usually at speed, the drag they created would pick me up off my feet, dropping me down again sometimes in the road. It was pretty scary. Kansas is famously the setting of *The Wizard of Oz*, and I often felt like Dorothy being swept up in a tornado. I just wished I had some ruby slippers so I could click my heels and be in New York!

As well as having the strong winds to contend with, the rain often tipped down in Kansas. So much so that we experienced more flash flooding, forcing us to change my route, adding additional miles. It wasn't just the weather, the terrain and my aches and pains that made Kansas my least favourite state so far. It was here that we encountered an angry troll on the morning of the twenty-third day. The crew had kept it quiet from me, but a critical discussion had been started on a popular American running forum, questioning my integrity during the challenge. At many points we were in the middle of nowhere, so we didn't have a mobile phone signal and Wi-Fi coverage. This meant we weren't always able to upload my stats online instantly. Another issue was that one of the trackers needed a 4G mobile signal in order to work, and often we couldn't get more than 3G. This had raised suspicion from some of those following my progress, particularly those who were enjoying the "race" for the world record between Sandra and I, and were hoping she would win.

Jenny had managed to arrange a new tracker to be brought out by Tim, and she was frequently travelling long distances to towns off our route in one of the support cars so she could find places like cafes with free Wi-Fi to upload my details and explain the delay. But still questions kept being asked. The crew were doing everything they could to ensure every mile and stop I made was covered and were trying to update my social media accounts as much as possible with pictures, live videos and information on my progress. We had a constant stream of witnesses, plus the film crew accompanying me getting lots of footage. But one member of the forum was so keen to prove I must have been cheating, he apparently drove for more than 5 hours to ambush us (the tracker was working well enough then for him to find me).

Usually I welcomed the company of people who were able to join me thanks to following my progress via the tracker. The people I had met so far along my way were really lifting my spirits, and I was often overwhelmed by their generosity and kindness. Unfortunately, this guy wanted to stalk rather than support me, and he did so in quite a dangerous way. Being a member of the police force, Jan was more attuned to this type of thing than the rest of us, and she first noticed him about 15 minutes after I set off running with Sophie that morning. It wasn't long until Sophie noticed him too.

"It looks like we have a car following us," she observed with concern. I tried not to worry about it, but as the morning went on, he was still there, constantly driving slowly a slight distance behind us like a lioness creeping up on her prey. Jenny and Tim decided they should speak to him but every time one of the support cars tried to get near him, he would drive off at full speed, whizzing past me with seemingly no regard for my safety. Later, he would then pop up behind us again. It was getting extremely creepy but also reckless. Often, he would get in the way of other road users as he was travelling at a snail's pace while also holding his mobile phone up while driving to film me. Drivers stuck behind him would have to overtake and accelerate past him and then me, many of whom wouldn't have been aware I was there until they were upon me. It was adding extra stress on what was already a scary section of road for me, thanks to the lack of a hard shoulder. In the end, Jan said we should call the police. They soon arrived, pulled him over and gave him a warning, so thankfully he didn't bother us again. Apparently he told them he thought I was cheating because the water bottles I was carrying in my vest were rocket propellers!

Sadly this encounter exposed me to the negative side of social media. I knew that by doing a world record attempt, quite rightly people would want to know I was doing everything properly. I have previously had three world records ratified by Guinness with every "i" dotted and every "t" crossed to produce a huge document of evidence, so I know how to do it by the book. The crew and I were making sure we stuck to all of Guinness' rules and we were using technology as best as we could to aid the documentation of my journey.

Despite this, and my proven track record of success, I still received some of the most outrageous abuse and nasty comments online. Some of this was highly personal and hurtful. While some of these trolls posted in forums and on social network sites, others went as far as personally sending me abusive emails. These were all intercepted by Jenny, so I was shielded from them at the time.

Tim was also getting messages from concerned friends at home warning him the internet was alive with chatter because not all our trackers were working correctly. Tim found this frustrating, as the trackers were for my and the crew's benefit and so people could follow me online; they weren't designed to be part of the evidence for the world record. Again, he didn't share any of this with me at the time, but when I was back home in the UK after the challenge, hearing and reading about it all was shocking and made my blood boil. None of the vitriol was coming from anyone in Sandra's camp and her coach, Dave Krupski, had messaged me at the time to say they didn't agree with the accusations being made by her fans.

He wrote: "I just wanted to say ALL of us in Sandra's camp FULLY believe Mimi is running an honest transcon [transcontinental] and we hope she has the best run possible! Of course we want Sandra to win, but that doesn't mean we can't root for Mimi to have the best run possible as well."

He added that we should take Taylor Swift's advice when it comes to dealing with haters and doubters and "Shake It Off".

I didn't read any of these comments at the time. Once I was home and started to catch up on a few, I knew Dave was right, and I shouldn't pay attention to the trolls. I made the decision not to read all of the negative comments and abusive emails I had been sent, as I knew it wouldn't be good for me. Tim agreed that I was better off ignoring it.

"It is just a shame none of them offered to run with you or to join us for a day or so to witness what was actually going on," he said.

Although I wasn't enjoying my time running through Kansas, there was a major highlight on day 25, as we reached the halfway point, having covered a distance of 1,425 miles (2,293 km). At the time, I had no idea where we were in terms of total distance – I just concentrated on one day at a time. It was the crew who totted up the mileage, writing everything down. As I ran towards my lunch stop, I was confused when I saw the RV covered in pink balloons and I wondered what they were for. I burst into tears when the crew revealed we were exactly halfway, and the pink balloons were to mark the milestone.

There was then another surprise in store for me as we toasted reaching halfway with sparkling apple juice (we know how to party!). Tim announced he wasn't going to be flying home as I had expected; he was going to stay till the end. I had been dreading him flying back home from Kansas as originally planned, as I knew I was really going to miss him. I needed his support more than ever to get to New York. I was so overjoyed when he told me he had always intended to stay for the rest of the record attempt but had decided not to mention it so he could surprise me. I gave him a huge hug and burst into more tears. It was very emotional. Everyone else had known all along that Tim was going to stay and loved seeing my reaction to the news.

"That was such a beautiful moment," Susie gushed. "It was like a proposal!" She added: "I'm glad the secret is now out as I'd noticed you were starting to wilt a little at the prospect of Tim leaving. You two are like teenagers in love. It's clear to see his presence really lifts you up and keeps you going."

She was right and I set off on my afternoon run feeling invigorated. Not only was I delighted Tim was staying, I knew it was a massive achievement to have made it halfway across the continent, and I had done it in the time frame I had planned. If I could do the same again, I would be in New York in another 25 days' time, after 50 days of running, well inside the current record. I knew I couldn't think that far ahead, as thinking about the distance still to go was overwhelming, so I continued putting one foot in front of the other, taking one day at a time. I was on track for the record, but there was still a very long way to go and my body was really starting to feel the strain.

This was evident on day 27 of the run when I felt for the first time that I couldn't complete my target daily miles. I managed to run 31.14 miles (50.11 km) before lunch but then I just couldn't face carrying on to do the afternoon stint. I was exhausted. Jenny quite rightly said that from a psychological point of view, it would be better if I did at least a further 10 miles (16 km) to take my daily total over 40 miles (64 km). This would also give the crew time to find a suitable place to stop for the night, as our lunchtime location was unsuitable for a long stay. I managed to drag myself out followed by a support car while the remaining crew went on ahead 10 miles (16 km) to find somewhere we could park for the night. Once I reached them, I was relieved to be stopping but disappointed with myself for not being able to go further that afternoon. But I knew it was the right decision. Extra rest at this point was important to keep my body going.

The following day I felt much more refreshed, so I tried not to dwell on the fact I hadn't completed my target miles the day before. Sophie was running with me and reminded me I had still managed to clock up over 40 miles (64 km) on what I felt had been a bad day. We were passing through Emporia at around 7 a.m. when we spotted a red car just ahead of us with a guy standing next to it. As we got closer, he called across asking if I was Mimi. I replied that yes I was, and he said he was on his way to work but had followed my tracker and wanted to come and say hello. After chatting for a bit, I realized he was the man who had first exposed a British ultrarunner for cheating when he claimed to have run a world record across America. Perhaps he was checking that I wasn't cheating after seeing all those comments from the online trolls, who knows. What I did know as we approached the next state line was that I would be pleased to leave Kansas behind.

CHAPTER FOUR

PAIN, PAIN, GO AWAY...

5–10 OCTOBER
STATE SEVEN: MISSOURI
DISTANCE COVERED: 282.10 MILES (454 KM)
DREXEL TO MISSISSIPPI RIVER, ALTON

We all instantly fell in love with Missouri. The people there were so incredibly warm, friendly and generous. The scenery was beautiful too. Jan was spot on when she described it as "very much like England, but on a much bigger scale." The countryside all around us looked very similar to that at home. There was no state line sign to pose beside for photos when we entered on the afternoon of the twenty-ninth day of the run, but simply a T-junction and a road called State Line Road to denote we were now in our seventh state.

It was a relief to be running on a wonderfully empty, virtually traffic-free road, allowing me the time to take in the beautiful scenery around me. It felt very remote with fields as far as you could see. I was enjoying the peace and quiet when all of a sudden in the distance behind me I could hear a loud rumbling sound getting closer and closer.

What is that racket? I thought, annoyed that it was disturbing what was a beautiful and quiet moment. Soon it became clear it was a car hurtling towards me. As it overtook, I saw two friendly guys inside a customized 1950s classic Cadillac waving as they drove by. They drove on for a bit then turned around to stop just ahead of me, getting out of their car to introduce themselves. They had encountered some of the crew further back on the road and had stopped to ask them what they were doing before catching up with me. They were called Noah and Mitchell and were real-life cowboys! They were delightful company and when I had to carry on running, they promised they would be back to see me again with a surprise.

The following morning, having had my ankle strapped as it was sore when I set out to run at 5 a.m., lo and behold they were waiting with coffee and cinnamon buns for everyone. They had actually arrived at 4 a.m. but waited in their vehicles until they saw us come out of Monty. They knew the owner of a local coffee shop/restaurant in the nearby town of Archie who had opened up early to provide us with the delicious freshly baked buns. I was so grateful but sadly I had to get running straight away to stay on schedule. As much as I would have liked to have been able to stop and chat to the people who visited me for longer, I was running against the clock and Sandra and, for all I knew, it could come down to minutes or even seconds between us over who got the record. Plus, as delicious as they looked and smelled, I knew eating pastries and then running doesn't mix for me. They would have sat heavily in my stomach and made me feel nauseous or given me a stitch. The crew, however, were thrilled and we were all extremely touched by their generosity. Jan and Tim were then lucky enough to be given a free breakfast at the restaurant when they stopped to refuel the RV at a garage that happened to be right beside it.

Meanwhile, as Sophie and I ran through Archie in the dark with our head torches on, we suddenly saw lots of people lining the streets waving and clapping with whoops of encouragement. Once again, I was bowled over by the kindness of strangers and it reinstated my faith in people after the unpleasant encounter in Kansas. It was such a lovely thing for them to do for a complete stranger so early in the morning, and certainly brightened up the start of what was to be a very wet, rainy day.

After lunch I finally reached the Katy Trail, a part of the route I had been really looking forward to since I started planning the run across America. It was once a railway line with trains running between Missouri, Kansas and Texas. Now the 240-mile (386-km) stretch has been converted into a recreational trail which is beloved by ramblers, runners and cyclists. It is the ideal place to enjoy the great outdoors as it is surrounded by beautiful woodland and filled with wildlife. It intersects the Missouri River so at times you are running alongside it, and at others crossing bridges over it, or passing under it through former railway tunnels.

I was excited about finally having a long stint running away from traffic-filled roads on this flat, scenic path. However, running along the trail as darkness fell turned a pleasant situation into something more hazardous as it became harder to see the path in front of me. The ground was covered with large conker-like objects that had fallen from some of the overhanging branches, making it very easy to ruin my ankle if I landed on one, so I had to really watch my footing. My left ankle, which had flared up while running on the off-road terrain in Arizona, became a concern again, but by now I had so many aches and pains, especially in my right leg, that it was just another one to try to block out.

I relished the peace and quiet of the trail. First thing in the morning, it was a joy to have it to ourselves and be off the busy roads. It was lovely to see the occasional runner or cyclist who went past me, most of them offering a cheery "hi". A group of ladies from Archie joined me for a few hours in the afternoon and their cheerful chatter took my mind off the pain.

Listening to their stories was fascinating but I was shocked when one told me she was carrying a loaded pistol. She said she always took one running with her, as otherwise she didn't feel safe. I often go out on training runs alone in the countryside where I live and I am grateful I never feel the need to take a weapon with me. I know there is a different attitude in America to guns, but I would be terrified and extremely uncomfortable about handling one, and it's certainly not part of my essential running kit!

Having said goodbye, I continued on my own until I met up with the crew a few miles further on. After a quick bite to eat, I was then joined by a delightful young man called Tyler who accompanied me for about 2 miles, again full of chatter. He was only 13 and every weekend would come to Calhoun County to stay with his grandparents, who lived off the Katy Trail. He would work at a chicken farm so he could give the money to his grandparents for his keep. It was really special to meet him and learn about his life and plans for the future, and I have no doubt he will achieve his dreams.

Day 31 of the run was certainly one to celebrate as it was Sophie's twenty-fifth birthday. Sadly we didn't have any bubbles to toast her with but we did have cake! The day began with Sophie and I running 10 miles (16 km) together, as usual chatting about nothing in particular but it was always good to talk.

Before my lunch break when I was alone again, my Garmin led me up a dirt track that I didn't realize was the wrong way until I had run about a mile. I was then desperate for a drink and knew I was now an extra mile away from getting one. I also felt a bit flustered and annoyed that I was wasting time going back on myself. Thankfully the film crew again saved the day as they had seen the path I took and followed me. Once they caught up with me, they gave me some water and rang the crew to tell them what had happened so they knew I would be at the next stop later than planned and wouldn't panic. It was another occasion when I was so glad that I had agreed to Carol and Susie joining us. As Carol had predicted, throughout the trip we did forget they were there in terms of feeling self-conscious about being filmed, but she and Susie also became indispensable members of the team and were generally just good company.

That afternoon, I had a scary encounter with a pack of four dogs. I'm used to attracting the attention of dogs when I am running. Usually they are just curious and playful but one in this pack was particularly vicious. I was running through a rural area when they suddenly charged at me as I ran past a house. Their owner seemed completely unconcerned and did nothing to call them back. One was snarling and jumping up at me while showing his teeth.

I am not scared of dogs and I usually find shouting a firm "no!" causes them to leave me alone. But this one wasn't giving up. The owner appeared to have absolutely no control over it and kept shouting at me to get into the support car that was following me at the time in order to get away from it. My crew tried to explain to her what I was doing and that if I got into a moving car I would be breaking the rules set out by Guinness. Instead, Tim drove the vehicle slowly so I could run with the car between myself and the persistent dog.

As we turned a corner further up the dirt road, we all thought it was safe, but unfortunately the dog then charged down the road towards me again; I have never seen a dog looking so angry. This time it was even more determined, jumping up and biting my right leg. Luckily, I had so much tape on it didn't penetrate the skin, but it did cause a bruise. There was no apology from the owner; it seemed as though she didn't care. I appreciate that she probably didn't have anyone running by her house very often because it was in such a remote location, and that the dogs were guarding their property, but it was pretty frightening being chased by the pack.

While that was a moment on the trip I would rather forget, there were others that will remain banked in my memory for the rest of my life. One of these moments came in Missouri when I was running towards Versailles. After my lunch break, horse-drawn carriages started overtaking me. On board I could see Amish people in their traditional dress. It made such a change from seeing vehicles on the roads and made me feel as though I had stepped back in time.

Horse-drawn carriage after carriage whizzed by. There were so many, I assumed they must be on their way to a gathering of some sort. I was amazed at how fast their horses could go and envied their speed and finesse as I was getting increasingly slower. Later, when darkness fell at around 8 p.m. and I had only my head torch for illumination, I encountered them again when I saw the road ahead was lit up by twinkling, flashing lights coming towards me. As the Amish carriages went past it was a sight to behold, as each one had strings of fairy lights wrapped around it – even the horses had lights on. It was a truly magical moment.

It was good to have distractions like this as the pain in my right leg was getting worse and worse. Sometimes it was a tightness in my hamstring and other times I felt like all the muscles in my leg were pulling in all the wrong directions. By this stage, even lying down and trying to get to sleep was becoming painful, and turning over from my stomach to my back would cause shooting pains to go up and down the back of my right leg. I tried my best to ignore it, knowing that in the morning I had to get up and run more than 50 miles (80 km). I had to get to New York.

Despite the discomfort I was in overnight, I was somehow managing to wake up each morning feeling positive and not tired. I was always able to get up and run. And I never doubted my ability to be able to finish what I had set out to do. But I did start to question how I was going to cope with the increasing pain levels. Some days everything flowed and I felt I was running well and my body was strong; other days my right leg was making me feel frustrated and cross. It was as though my body was running two different events. My left leg was happy and didn't feel as though it had done anything more than a marathon, whereas my right leg could feel every step of the 1,500-plus miles (2,400-plus km).

With the pain increasing I subconsciously tried not to put too much pressure on my right side, resulting in my body tilting towards the left. I wasn't aware of this until my crew pointed it out.

"You look like you may topple over at any moment," Tim told me. I didn't believe him until he showed me a photo and he was right. I looked ridiculous. No wonder I was starting to have an issue with my back too.

"Hopefully a massage will sort me out and it won't be as bad tomorrow," I said optimistically.

Unfortunately, this was another day I was having to go longer between treatments as physiotherapist Beccy was due to fly home. Jenny would drive her to the airport and would then have to wait to collect her replacement Nicola from her flight. I wouldn't be able to have a massage until Nicola arrived, hopefully by the time of my lunchtime stop. Before she left, I thanked Beccy for all her hard work. I was flattered when she said she had been amazed by my pain threshold and determination and I was glad to hear she had enjoyed the experience.

"It has been a great way to travel across the US, especially being able to talk to voters ahead of the presidential elections," she said. "I feel I have experienced authentic America."

As well as observing my running style, Tim had also been busy map reading – something he is very good at. As we approached Jefferson City the following day, he found a path that was more direct than our intended route. He said he would join me to follow it as it wasn't straightforward. It made my life much easier having someone there to navigate and it was lovely having my husband for company. Fittingly, we ran together across the Jefferson City Bridge that goes over the Missouri River, as it is a popular spot for love birds. It was lined with thousands of padlocks that have been attached to the railings. Known as "love locks", they symbolize a couple's love for one another and usually have names or initials engraved onto them. A couple will attach theirs, and then throw the key into the river to represent their unbreakable love. Tim and I didn't have the foresight or time to attach our own, but I think spending so much time together in tough conditions doing the world record attempt was enough to represent our unbreakable love!

Coming off the very tall bridge, we had to spiral down a walkway four times until we reached a park at the bottom. This pedestrianized walkway from the bridge had been created to give more people access to the Katy Trail, which we were about to join again. Anyone looking at the path we took on my Garmin map afterwards must have thought we had got lost and were going around in circles as our path looped like a tornado as we descended from the bridge. In fact, we did get a little bit lost when we reached the ground, as we came to a section under the bridge which was very overgrown. It was hard to find the path we were supposed to be following and I started to get a bit annoyed at this point. I was tired and just wanted to reunite with the rest of the crew, have my lunch and a massage before continuing with the second half of the day. It was just as well Tim was with me as he soon had us back on track and we reached the RV without further delay.

After lunch, I meandered along the Katy Trail for the remainder of the day and most of the following morning with occasional views of the Missouri River. For the first time on the trip, that morning we had overslept. Jan always set her alarm for 4.30 a.m. so she could be up first to start making breakfast for me and the crew and wake everyone else up. On this occasion her alarm didn't go off and she woke with a start at 4.50 a.m. You would have thought I would have enjoyed a lie-in but I had actually been wide awake lying in bed waiting to hear her alarm. Once we realized what had happened, I was up and dressed, drank as much of my breakfast smoothie as I could (the remainder was put into my water bottle to have as I ran) and I set off only 3 minutes later than usual so it wasn't a disaster. Jan felt awful but quite rightly pointed out it was unfair the wake-up call was always her responsibility. She asked the rest of the crew to remember to set their alarms too from now on.

As I carried on through Missouri, I tried my best to take my mind off the pain I was now in and just focus on ticking off each mile – another mile run was another one closer to finishing. Leaving the Katy Trail behind to run on a road towards Case was a bit of a shock to the system. Although the surface was easier to run on, it meant having to cope once again with lorries and cars storming past in a hurry to get to their destination. I often feared for my safety when they sped by without always leaving much space between them and me. Then I realized I wasn't the only one in danger when I saw something crawling slowly across the road ahead of me. When I got closer, I noticed it was a tortoise. I knew I couldn't just leave it where it was as it was heading very slowly into the middle of the road and it was likely to be flattened before it made it across. I carefully picked it up and then placed it further away from the road to continue its journey. My good deed done for the day.

Soon I felt as though I was moving as slowly as the tortoise had been. At times I had to power walk instead of run to give myself a bit of respite from the pain in my leg and back. One of these power walking sections coincided with a guy called Brian joining me. He had heard about my world record attempt from the podcast *Marathon Talk* and decided to come and run with me from Pendleton to Warrenton. It was lovely to meet him and I felt grateful for his company for a few miles that day. He must have been disappointed that I couldn't run at that point as it was too painful. He returned the next day and this time we did do some running together, his company helping to put a spring back in my step.

The lunch stop on this day was on the edge of Graus Lake, about 18 miles (29 km) from the Illinois border. Tim, being a fly fisherman, was beside himself with excitement because Jenny had bought him a toy fishing rod from Walmart to play with. He attached a piece of ham to the end of the rod and sat by the lake with great anticipation waiting for a fish. By the time I arrived still nothing had been caught!

The afternoon weather provided a welcome distraction from my aches and pains as I ran: the most spectacular storm started to take place around me. The sky darkened with black clouds and then rumbled with thunder. When I looked at the gathering of clouds off to my right, I could see them lit up with flashing lightning bolts. It was very dramatic, an entertaining light show put on by Mother Nature. When the thunderstorm died down, then came gale-force winds. The lorries that drove by now seemed to be struggling to stay upright, so you can imagine how difficult it was for me, particularly with my lopsided running style.

Just keep moving forward, I told myself.

Tim drove to find me towards the end of the wet and windy 10 miles (16 km) with some hot noodles. I carried on making step after painful step. I was making progress. It was slow progress, but Tim reassured me that didn't matter.

"You are so far ahead of the record, even if you have to walk the rest of the way, you will still get it," he told me. While that was a bit of an exaggeration, he was right in that I was still covering the ground and getting closer to my destination, even if I wasn't going as fast as I had been before.

In the early evening of 10 October, day 34 of my run across America, Tim and I crossed over the mighty Mississippi River via Clark Bridge. This incredible cable-stayed bridge is 1,408 m (4,620 feet) long and I marvelled at how impressive it is. Although there was a wide enough space for me to run along it away from the vehicles, I was being blown in all directions and felt very vulnerable because of the incredibly strong winds. I couldn't stop to look at the river for fear of being blown off the bridge, but I knew I had to take in some of this milestone moment. Not only is the river one of the country's most famous natural wonders, but also once halfway across it, I would pass into my eighth state, Illinois, the Land of Lincoln.

10–13 OCTOBER
STATE EIGHT: ILLINOIS
DISTANCE COVERED: 156.16 MILES (251.32 KM)
MIDDLE OF THE MISSISSIPPI RIVER, ALTON TO EAST OF MARSHALL

Day 35 started off badly. I had only been running for about a mile when I needed to take a short break so Nicola could work her magic on my leg and give me some more tape. I didn't know if the taping would make any difference, but it was the only option I seemed to have. Thankfully it did the trick and I managed to get some good miles in that morning, joined by Jan for a few of them.

I clocked up just over 30 miles (48 km), using all my usual tactics to try to alleviate the pain so I could keep moving forwards. I listened to music which helped for a time and when the healing property of the music wore off, I tried to empty my mind of everything, which is another method that usually helps. I focus on the here and now, literally what is in front of me, and putting one foot in front of the other. I don't think of the miles I have done, or the miles I have yet to do. Even the scenery takes a back seat as it is too hard to process it. I simply stay in the present – in that moment. This usually works well for me but this time the pain I was now experiencing was on another level to anything I had felt before. Trying to clear my mind was a real struggle as my body was screaming at me to stop so I could get rid of the excruciating pain. But I couldn't stop; I had to find another way to cope.

Focusing on my family was usually another thing that helped. I had a picture of them in my mind all standing at the finish line in New York waiting for me to run up the steps in triumph and give them a big hug. But even this only provided very brief respite. When I stopped for lunch, I could see concern on all the faces of the crew. I didn't have to tell them how much pain I was in. They could see it by the way I was moving, the gritted expression on my face, and the occasional wail I made when my right foot hit the ground.

"I've tried everything," I told them. "I don't know what I can do to make this more bearable. I have never felt pain like this before."

"I think you need to see a doctor," Jenny said.

I agreed in the hope they would have a miracle solution to allow me to carry on running without being in so much agony. As luck would have it, my route that afternoon was going to go straight past a hospital. Jenny rang ahead to check whether I needed an appointment, but we were told just to come in as it was very quiet.

Once there, I was seen immediately and given an X-ray. They couldn't find a specific problem with my bones but pointed out the obvious – I was suffering because of all the miles I had run. They did offer me some painkillers, but I had to be careful which ones I took. I couldn't take anything during the record attempt that would be deemed performance-enhancing, and many painkillers are not safe to take when exercising. So what I was able to take didn't really make much difference.

I left the hospital feeling frustrated and fed up. I knew they couldn't "cure" me of all the agony I was in. I just wanted them to be able to fix me in some way so I could carry on with a manageable level of pain. I had no choice but to power walk the afternoon section. To my delight, Tim walked with me for the last 2 miles of the day. I managed 16.33 miles (26.28 km) bringing my daily total to 48.01 miles (77.26 km). This was the second time I had run fewer than 50 miles (80 km) in a day since the run had started. I wanted to scream and shout and get angry. I was cross with my body as I felt it was letting me down. But I knew getting mad wouldn't help or achieve anything. As the saying goes, I had to keep calm and carry on.

I could see my despondency was having a knock-on effect on the crew too as the atmosphere among them had changed. I thrive off positivity and I needed them to help pick me up when I was feeling low. When I finished that evening, the crew had to help me up the steps of the RV due to the pain. Suddenly I felt as though I was about 90 years old. I really needed a morale boost, but they obviously didn't know what to say to be encouraging. Their silence was ominous. Had they given up on me already? Of course not, and when I reached the bedroom I saw they had found a way to make me feel better. Sophie had come up with the brilliant idea of hanging up a map of America on the back wall of my room. She had marked on it the route we had taken with various comments of funny events that had happened along the way, such as where accident-prone Tim had lost the RV awning, where we had encountered the tarantulas and where we had met the marvellous cowboys. It was just the tonic I needed, and I burst into tears.

Thankfully the next day I felt much better after getting a good night's sleep. I was delighted during my morning run when Jim McCord came to see me. He has run across America himself and looks after a Facebook page called USA Crossers that keeps a record of everyone who attempts the journey. He joined me for a few miles of power walking while also broadcasting a live interview with me via Facebook. It was wonderful to chat about the sights I had seen during my journey so far and he asked me to describe the ways I was trying to deal with the pain. I was very flattered when he told people tuning in that I have the best personality of all the runners he has ever met, and he had no doubt I would make it to New York. I could have done without him constantly reminding people of my age though. "Mimi is fifty-five years old!!!" he declared more than once. I was grateful he took the time out to see me and it was a real boost chatting to him and the outside world after feeling so low the day before.

Another much-needed boost was reaching the 2,000-mile (3,219-km) mark, meaning I had fewer than 900 miles (1,448 km) to go to reach New York. As I arrived at the support vehicle Nicola and Jan started singing in celebration. It was an incredibly emotional moment, but I was too focused on getting the miles in for the rest of the day to cry as I would normally do! Spirits were high among us all again and I managed to cover over 32 miles (51 km) before lunch.

In the afternoon, I received a wonderful, but rather random, act of kindness from a stranger who made me smile. I had been running along Route 40 for what seemed like an eternity. It was like Groundhog Day, on and on along the same stretch of road. It was very dull mentally and I was having my usual battle with the oncoming traffic. There was one particular lorry that was coming towards me that caused concern as it didn't look as though it was going to move out. It continued to get closer still, but eventually slowed down and then stopped right in front of me. Totally ignoring the cars queuing up behind him, the driver climbed down from his cab. I thought he was going to shout at me for being on the road but instead he handed me a can of V8 Juice (a vegetable smoothie) and said: "As the advert says, 'the best way to start your day!' I think what you are doing is fantastic." He then got back in his lorry and drove off, leaving me feeling much happier and grinning from ear to ear for miles after.

Meanwhile, Tim had the most difficult task of trying to find a spot to park the RV that night. As permission was always needed, it was often tricky to find somewhere with enough space, where it also wouldn't be too noisy and disturb our sleep. In some places it was really difficult to gain permission because we could be many miles from the nearest habitation, or in a small town with no sign of people. Tim would often joke that everyone must have been "spirited away by aliens" as he could go for miles driving the RV in semi-suburban areas and never see another soul.

On this occasion, he had found the only possible parking spot with a dusty drive leading up to a house about 100 yards further up the track. He parked the RV and walked up to the house to seek permission to park there. After ringing the doorbell and knocking on the door, he waited for a response but there was only silence. He walked around to the side of the house and could see through a window that lights were on and the fridge door was open. The house was very definitely lived in as he could see milk and other fresh contents in the fridge.

He called out "Hello?" and knocked on the window, putting his face up against the glass to see inside better. Still getting no response he gave up and walked back down the track towards the RV. Halfway there, he saw a police car with its lights flashing racing towards him and wondered what had occurred. It pulled over when it reached him, and the local Sheriff stepped out with his hand hovering over his holster. Tim admitted he wasn't as concerned as he should have been as he knew he hadn't committed any crime and was actually finding the situation quite amusing. The Sheriff was not amused though.

"Have you been to that house?" he asked him, pointing to the home Tim had been knocking at. When Tim explained he had and why, the Sheriff told him a terrified Mexican maid was inside and had called him for help.

"She told me a rough-looking man was trying to break into the house," he said. "She's been hiding under the kitchen table and was particularly scared when you pressed your face to the window."

Tim was mortified he had caused such a reaction.

"I must say when I saw my unkempt hair and bearded face in the wing mirror of the RV, I am not surprised she was scared," he told me later.

Needless to say, once all had been explained, we were given permission to park there, which was a relief, and hearing Tim's experience did make me laugh.

I continued on Route 40 for the whole of the next day. Although I was bored of running on the same stretch of road, it made navigation easy. It was often favourable to going through towns too. I dreaded passing through built-up areas as it would really slow my progress. I did go through some beautiful towns, some really olde worlde places that seemed untouched by time and looked like a Western film set. Unfortunately, sometimes it looked like the pavements hadn't been touched for decades either. I found they were very inadequately maintained, I suppose because the Americans in general tend to drive more than walk to places, even when travelling short distances. The paving slabs were so uneven I worried about tripping or turning over on my ankle.

There was one town in Illinois I was delighted to run through though, as it was beautifully quirky. Casey bills itself as "a small town with big ideas". Everything you pass is larger than life. It is home to the world's largest rocking chair, wind chime and post box among other giant items. It was the brainchild of a local man called Jim Bolin, who constructed the huge installations with the help of his crew, putting his town on the map in the process. Tourists flock to see the super-sized objects and I made time to stop and have my picture taken beside some of them as this was not something you saw every day.

I then reached one particular section of road on the way towards Terre Haute which was incredibly dangerous to run on. It was getting dark and the traffic was heavy and speeding past me. There was no hard shoulder and no space to get off the road if I needed to because a large barrier stretched alongside it. Tim met me at the crossroads and told me that they had decided to proceed with one of the support cars driving behind me like an escort. I was so tired that at first I misunderstood. I thought he was saying I would have to get into the car and be driven along this section.

"Don't be ridiculous, I can't do that," I told him. "It would be cheating. The rules state I can't do any of the route in a moving vehicle."

He laughed and clarified: "No, you run, and we will drive behind you for safety."

This turned out to be a marvellous idea. It was the safest I had felt while running for days. I ran in the direction of the traffic, instead of against it which is what I usually did unless there was a wide hard shoulder, while Tim trailed me with the car lights flashing. Finishing my run each day continued to be a huge relief but I found the overnight rest wasn't giving me much respite from the pain. I dreaded waking up at around 2 a.m. bursting for a pee, as I knew it would be a challenge to go to the loo. I had to ease down slowly from the bed, putting my right leg on the floor in an attempt to stand up. This would send shooting pains up my leg that were excruciating, causing me to cry out and worry I had woken one of the crew. As I couldn't put any pressure on my right leg, I would have to swivel my way out of my room using the walls for support, then hobble from my bedroom, grabbing onto the bunk beds (where Sophie and Darren were sleeping) for more support to reach the RV toilet/shower room, all while trying to be as quiet as possible. I would then have to haul myself through the narrow cubicle door, gritting my teeth with the pain, and swivel with great difficulty to turn and sit on the loo.

It was amazing how an act I usually took for granted had become such a hardship. As I sat on the loo relieved to have made it, I would hold my head in my hands wondering how on earth I was going to get out of bed in just over 2 hours' time and persuade my body to run 50-something miles again. But that was thinking too far ahead, as first I had to drag myself from the shower room to make it back to bed.

* * *

There are moments when I'm running when my wonderful father pops into my head for a chat. One particular morning while I was running through Illinois, a picture of him appeared in my mind. He passed away in 2007 of bladder cancer and I miss him terribly. He was always incredibly supportive of my running – although I think he was slightly surprised as I had never been a runner at school, preferring to play team sports.

I hope you're proud of me, Dad. I always knew this was going to be a hard challenge to take on. I'm beginning to really struggle with the pain but whatever happens I know you are here with me, I am going to finish and I'm not ready to give up yet, I told him.

I knew he would have been proud of me. He always encouraged me to chase my dreams and taught me to believe nothing is impossible. The very last conversation I had with him was along these lines. I had been due to compete in the 6633 Arctic Ultra when we were told he didn't have long to live. I was going to cancel the trip, but he insisted I go. He wanted me to take on the extraordinary challenge of running 352 miles (566 km) in the Arctic because his cancer proved life is too short not to pursue your goals. With his and the rest of my family's blessing, I went. I was devastated to learn when I finished that he passed away when I was halfway through the eight-day race. It will sound strange, but I believe I felt the moment he passed away. I had been running along the long ice road, which was actually the frozen-over Mackenzie River, when I suddenly felt like I had been punched in the heart and I couldn't breathe. A huge sense of loss overwhelmed me. Somehow, I just knew my father had died. It was as if I could feel his presence, as though he had come to see me to tell me himself. I couldn't give in to my grief then as I still had a solitary 120 miles (193 km) to run through the snowy wilderness. But thinking about my father and how I could do him proud spurred me on in the freezing conditions. I finished first overall, setting a new course record in the process. I knew he would have been incredibly proud of me and now I hoped I could make him proud again by reaching New York in world record time.

After nearly three days of running through Illinois, almost all on Route 40, I was relieved to reach the next state line to pass into Indiana. We were pretty much in the middle of nowhere at this point. There was no state sign, so Sophie made her own. She stood at the side of the road together with Jan and waved her "Welcome to Indiana" sign on cardboard at me as I ran past. I loved it but as I was now approaching the end of the day, I was in a lot of pain so could barely muster a smile. I just wanted to finish.

Indiana is known as the "Crossroads of America" but unfortunately it was going to be the end of the road for me. I didn't know it when I crossed into the state – pained but still determined to continue – but this would be the last one on my journey.

13–16 OCTOBER
STATE NINE: INDIANA
DISTANCE COVERED: 131.28MILES (211.27 KM)
EAST OF MARSHALL TO WEST OF CAMBRIDGE CITY

Passing into Indiana meant another time zone (Eastern) and another hour of lost sleep. I really felt this one. After running for the past 37 days, I was exhausted, and I needed as much rest as possible. It was Friday the thirteenth when I ran into Indiana and I thought I had done well to get through the day without any major mishaps. However, when I reached the RV for the night, I took off my top to have a shower and was dismayed to find something missing. I always ran with a brooch on my crop top that my godmother had given to me on the day I was christened. It was my lucky charm and had travelled the world with me. It must have fallen off somewhere along the 57.7 miles (92.9 km) I had run that day. I was gutted but I knew I couldn't dwell on it and I didn't have the energy to get upset about it. I knew we didn't have time to retrace our steps and it wasn't very big so it would be impossible to find. My only consolation was hoping that perhaps someone else might find it one day and treasure it as I had done. Hopefully it would bring them as much love and luck as it had brought me.

The next day, I tried to stick to our usual routine and reach my required morning miles but the pain in my right leg was now unbearable. To make matters worse, my back was incredibly sore due to my continued – and worsening – lean to the left. I looked like the Leaning Tower of Pisa. Far from the ideal running form. I was determined to carry on but after completing only 23 miles (37 km) that morning I knew my back needed urgent treatment to make this possible. Although Nicola was doing a great job as my physio, my back was so sore we decided it would be best if I saw a chiropractor. They specialize in manipulation of the spine and would have extra equipment to help me.

Once again, Jenny was amazing and rang around a few chiropractors to get me an appointment. Unfortunately, as it was a Saturday, many of them were closed, but she was finally able to book me an appointment in the afternoon with a chiropractor called Kevin who was also a fellow ultrarunner. We stopped at midday and staked out in accordance with the rules set out by Guinness so I could then be driven to my appointment. I don't remember much of the 45-minute journey as I slept in the back of the car after having eaten my lunch.

Kevin was amazing and gave me a full treatment. He massaged my back and gave me dry needle therapy on my legs, something I had never tried before, but it definitely helped. It was absolute heaven to be able to lie down on his couch. It was so relaxing, I found myself unable to keep my eyes open and I drifted off to sleep momentarily. Kevin kindly gave me a TENS machine and advised me to use it on my back muscles in the evenings. It is a device that sends small electrical impulses into your muscles that can reduce the pain signals between the spinal cord and brain. The impulses are believed to help relieve pain and relax muscles and help the body produce the feel-good hormones endorphins. Often women use them in childbirth to help ease labour pains. I had never used one before, so I thought it was worth a try. I later discovered it didn't make much difference to the pain I was in, which was definitely worse than childbirth in my experience.

I left the appointment feeling better and more optimistic again. Jenny and Nicola drove me back to where we had stopped a few hours earlier so I could resume running. The day had started so badly but I was back on the road again. It wasn't ideal that I had to have such a long break. The time I had spent at the chiropractors was all time added onto the record attempt. I could "stake out" to be allowed to attend the appointment via a car (at other times it was forbidden to be in a moving vehicle), but the clock didn't stop ticking.

I was now out of sync with my usual routine too, but as with any plan, I knew it was important to be adaptable at times. I still wasn't pain-free and the treatment on my body made me feel drained of energy so I ran-walked the remainder of the day, only covering 17.5 miles (28.2 km) in the afternoon, bringing my daily total to a mere 40.84 miles (65.73 km). I tried not to let this bother me as I was ahead of the schedule I had set myself, so a day of reduced mileage wasn't a disaster. However, it would be the last time I could do it as time was not on my side. I wasn't just running across America, this was a world record attempt. I needed to get my act together to do the fastest time possible. I couldn't afford to have any more short days.

I have somehow managed to get through today, so I will find a way of getting through the next day and the next... I told myself.

There was a surprise in store when I reached Monty for the night. To my delight, I had been paid a visit by the "second most famous" Santa in Indiana. It was only October, but he had heard about my run and wanted to share some festive spirit with us in advance of the big day. As you would expect of Father Christmas, he was very jolly and really cheered me up by stopping by to say hello. It was some very welcome light relief after what had been a difficult day.

Some of Santa's magic must have rubbed off on me as day 39 started surprisingly well after an extremely good night's sleep. The air was very humid and you could tell it was going to rain later. It was a relief to feel good as I felt under a huge amount of pressure to get some miles under my belt after the reduced mileage the day before. It was essential I covered the set distance of 57 miles (92 km) that day, otherwise my target would begin to slip away.

Jan and Nicola were in the support car looking after me in the morning while Sophie ran with me. When they parked up at a petrol station to wait for me, they were approached by a guy called James who asked them what I was doing and which charities I was raising money for. About an hour later, he reappeared further down the road and produced $400 in cash for the charities. I cried when the crew told me about it at my next stop.

"What a wonderful and generous thing to do!" I said. His generosity spurred me on, and I was pleased to reach 32.3 miles (51.98 km) before lunch. I was moving incredibly slowly but I had to accept that would be the case now I had run more than 2,000 miles. After lunch I was still in good spirits and I headed off for the final 25.7 miles (41.36 km) of the day. Finally, I finished at 9.30 p.m. having covered a glorious 58 miles (93.34 km). I had done it! I went to bed that night trying to stay positive despite how much pain my body was in.

Day 40 is one I would rather forget. I woke up twice in the night in a lot of pain. In the morning, my mind was still ready and willing to get up and run but my body wasn't having any of it. In the previous week, I had often found it difficult to get moving first thing as I felt so stiff, but once I had warmed up, things improved. Not today. Every step I took was causing shooting pains to go up and down my right leg and I felt seriously uncomfortable. Nicola suggested I try using the knee brace that the physios had told me to bring out in case I should need it. It was designed to "off load" my knee. I don't know why it hadn't been suggested I wear it before. It was too little, too late as it didn't make any difference now. My back and the whole of my right leg was in constant pain. I was groaning in agony every time my foot hit the ground. Darren was running with me and doing his very best to keep me motivated but nothing helped. Running simply wasn't an option. I was used to pushing myself to run through pain but this was unlike anything I had ever experienced before. I didn't know what to do. I stopped and burst into tears. I had tried everything and there was nothing that was helping make the pain bearable enough for me to continue. Nicola tried taping it in a different way but that didn't work. The pain was only getting worse.

After a good cry, I pulled myself together. I wasn't giving up yet. Every time I met up with the crew at the support car I begged for painkillers, which of course they wouldn't give me as I would have had an overdose with the amount I was asking for. I cried a lot, but the crew were amazing, continuing to motivate me to keep going forwards. I hobbled along but walking wasn't feeling much better than running. Each mile seemed to take longer and longer to complete.

The support car started waiting for me every mile and each time I saw them was another excuse to stop and take a break. I felt I was procrastinating but I needed to sit down and take the weight off my legs. Mile 14–15 took me over 25 minutes. When I met up with Tim and Nicola, once again they were very positive, but they could see how much pain I was in. There was no thought of stopping as far as I was concerned though. I knew I had to keep going as I couldn't keep having shorter days. Tim told me to keep moving as best as I could and he would talk to Jenny and decide what the next step would be.

This is ridiculous, I thought as I took step after agonizing step. *It's going to take me all day to cover a couple more miles at this rate*. I wondered what people who saw my Strava data would be thinking, probably that I had resorted to crawling. I wouldn't have even been able to manage that with the state my knees were in. I slowly made my way to where I was due to meet the crew at just under 16 miles (26 km).

"I can't carry on like this," I admitted. They all agreed. They hadn't let on to me, but they had spoken among themselves about how worried they were and how I couldn't continue as I was. Half of them went ahead to find a suitable spot to park the RV for the night. I then had to limp my way to join them so I could officially stake out.

Once in the RV, I had to finally acknowledge that my right knee was a serious issue. I had kept telling myself and the crew that it was fine and everything else around it was the problem, but I couldn't deny it any longer. I needed to know what was going on with the joint so I could then make a choice about how to deal with it and how to keep going. Jenny found a hospital in Richmond not far from where we had stopped where I would be able to go for an MRI scan. At this point, I had no doubt that I would return to this spot later and resume running. Yes, I had my concerns, but I thought this was just a blip, something that I could get sorted and then hit the road again. My plan was to have the scan, get the results, and then hopefully get some treatment. I hoped that additional painkillers or even a cortisone injection would allow me to keep running.

At the hospital, it was bliss to be taken to a bed and told to lie down. I was given some pain relief but informed I wouldn't be able to have my scan until the following morning. The delay wasn't ideal but I knew I had to stay positive. I needed this scan to be able to continue. If this time allowed me to find a way to carry on running with less pain, it would be worth it.

We had to return to the RV for the night where Jan cooked a lovely meal for Tim and me. I was a little put out when she and the rest of the crew announced they were all going to go out for dinner, leaving us behind. They probably wanted to give us some space and I completely understood that they needed a break and time away from the confinement of the RV. But as I was feeling so low at the time, I felt as though they had given up on me already and that they thought the world record attempt was over.

It felt strange waking up the next morning knowing I wasn't going to be getting up and going running as I had been for the past 40 days. I just wanted to get the scan done so I could be back on the road by the afternoon. At 5.30 a.m., Tim drove me to the hospital and the rest of the crew caught up with us later when the results were in. It was the worst possible news. The scan showed I had bone oedema, swelling at the back and on the medial side of my right knee. The cartilage had worn away so I was down to bone on bone on the lateral side of my knee. No wonder it had been so painful. Jenny looked at the scan and winced as the doctor explained how bad it was. I had tears rolling down my face as I tried to process what it all meant.

"Is there any way I can still run on it?" I asked him. The scan made that answer pretty obvious, but to his credit, the doctor never told me to stop running.

"It is your choice, it is your body," he told me. "But I have to warn you, you would be risking a number of serious injuries if you try to carry on running to New York. You are at risk of multiple stress fractures in your leg because your bones are considerably bruised. Your back, hips and legs could all suffer from stress fractures that it would take many months to recover from with complete rest. In your right knee, you are already rubbing bone on bone. The worst-case scenario if you continue is you will need a full knee replacement on returning home." He added: "I could give you a cortisone injection in the knee to try to continue, but that won't cure anything. It would only mask the pain for a short time, and it doesn't always work."

I considered the injection but wondered if it would be worth it. It might allow me to run for another two days – but I still had more than ten days and just over 600 miles (966 km) to go. It still wouldn't be enough to allow me to finish, and it would risk doing much greater long-term damage to my body. There was a high chance I would be unable to walk, let alone run for months if I didn't stop now.

I sat in shock, my face red and blotchy from all the crying. How had it come to this? I had heard all the facts, but I still wasn't ready to quit. I was desperately trying to think of ways to continue. Could I have multiple cortisone injections? Could I live with the consequences if I carried on? Was it worth risking further damage to have the record? Jenny told me she was going to leave me alone to think while she went to speak to the rest of the crew. She told them how serious my condition was and how much was at stake to my long-term health if I continued.

"She is still not willing to stop," she told them. "She wants to find a way to carry on."

"We have to make her see sense," Tim said. "The doctor told me he couldn't believe she thinks a few painkillers will solve this so she can be on her way. He has warned me I'll be taking her home in a wheelchair if she doesn't stop now, and the chances would be pretty high that she would need to have a knee replacement." He then told them: "I've always been in complete awe of what Mimi can do. I have seen her push through pain to succeed on many occasions, and I have often struggled to understand how her body can take the punishments she inflicts on it. But this time it is different. Seeing the way her knee is bending inwards with bone crunching on bone at every step is too difficult to watch. If she doesn't agree to stop, then for the first time in her running career, I am going to put my foot down and say I can't let her carry on. It is not safe. We wouldn't be doing our jobs as crew if we let her keep going."

They all agreed he was right, even though they were all as desperate to continue as I was.

"This is just heartbreaking," Sophie said. "Poor Mimi. I wish there was something we could do to help her."

It was decided Tim would be the best person to talk to me. They knew stopping was in my best interests, but it was me alone who had to make that final call. It was without a doubt the toughest decision of my life.

"I don't want to quit," I sobbed to Tim. I sat with my feet dangling over the edge of the couch, my hands covering my face as I rocked backwards and forwards sobbing uncontrollably. Deep down I knew there was only one choice. But I didn't want to give up; I still had my running kit on ready to go. I wanted to be driven back to where I had stopped and carry on running. I wanted to run to New York. I wanted to gain a new world record. But I had to look at the bigger picture. I didn't want to be taken home in a wheelchair and then be an invalid for months to come. I didn't want to go through knee replacement surgery; I was too young for that. I didn't want to keep running now and then never be able to run again for the rest of my life. While the thought of not being able to continue with the record attempt was soul-destroying, the thought of never being able to run in the future was even worse. I had a life after the world record, and I wanted running to be part of it. I was 55 years old and I still wanted to be running in not just a few years' time, but in 20 years' time. It didn't have to be far, but I knew just being able to go out and enjoy the trails would enhance the rest of my life.

It was my quality of life for the coming months and years I had to think about too. The damage I could cause to my body would be astronomical if I tried to keep running to New York. It just wouldn't be worth it. I knew no world record was worth my future long-term health and happiness.

"I'll stop," I told Tim in tears after an agonizing hour mulling it over. I felt as though I was letting down the crew, my supporters, and the charities I was running for. But I knew it was the right decision. I wanted to go on – but my body couldn't. I had run 2,215.24 miles (3,565.08 km) from California to Indiana in 40 days. I hadn't broken a world record, but I had nearly broken myself. It was time to call it a day before the damage to my body became irreversible. My run across America was over.

CHAPTER FIVE

FACING DEFEAT

With the decision made, it seemed (understandably) as though some of the crew just wanted to return to their usual lives as quickly as possible. We returned to the RV and Jenny went into overdrive, arranging and booking flights home for herself and the others at the earliest opportunity. There was a strange atmosphere; we were all finding it tough knowing how to handle the situation. For the past 40 days we had been following a routine where everyone knew what they were supposed to be doing. Suddenly everything had changed. I knew everyone was desperately disappointed and felt sad for me; I could tell a few of them had been crying. It was obvious they didn't know what they could say to make me feel better, so they didn't say much at all. Tim tried his best to console me and explain how the rest of the crew must be feeling.

"I have a terrible sense of sadness for you but perhaps also a tinge of selfish disappointment for myself," he admitted.

"We all wanted to be at the finish in New York and be part of this great record. We had all planned to be here for longer. Now we are left with a loss, a type of grief and thinking 'what now'?"

He apologized to me for feeling this way, and of course wasn't at all trying to make me feel bad. He was just trying to help me understand the sudden change in atmosphere and why the crew, who had been thinking of my needs for every waking moment for weeks, now didn't know what they could do for me.

"Everyone just feels a bit lost," he said. I felt the same way. This hadn't been part of the plan.

Instead of running the rest of the way to New York, we would have to drive. The following morning after Jenny had organized all the flights, we set off for New York. Tim and Jan took it in turns to drive the RV with me as a passenger. Darren, Jenny and Nicola travelled in one of the support cars, dropping Jenny off at the airport on the way, while Sophie drove the other support car with Tim and Jan taking it in turns to travel with her when they weren't driving the RV. Apparently Jan and Sophie had great fun singing "Country Roads" as they drove through West Virginia.

We drove to New York in one go, taking over 6 hours. With hindsight we should have broken up the journey as it was incredibly dangerous to drive that far on the little sleep the crew had all had, especially as it was on top of what had already been an exhausting few weeks. There was no need to have been in such a hurry, but perhaps everyone just wanted to get to New York and back home to their usual lives. I felt terrible being driven the final leg of my intended journey. I cried on and off for those 6 hours, struggling to come to terms with what had happened. We took the interstates so at least I didn't have to see the roads I would have run along.

RVs aren't allowed in Manhattan but I had found an RV park in Liberty Harbour, in sight of the Statue of Liberty, where we could stay. Trying to find it at around 9 p.m. was difficult but eventually we arrived, followed shortly by the support cars and the film crew's RV. Having parked up, we had some food and went to bed in the RV for the final time – we were exhausted. At around 4.30 a.m. the following morning, Sophie and Nicola were picked up by a cab to take them to the airport. We had said our goodbyes the evening before which had been very emotional after everything we had been through.

There was a lot of clearing up to do in the cars as well as the RV. It seemed such a waste to throw away the food we wouldn't eat and extra items like chairs we had bought for sitting outside on. Thankfully Carol and Susie, who were emptying their own RV, had found a local charity centre supporting women and children in need where we could donate everything. It made me feel better that something positive had come out of my negative experience.

It was then time for the remaining crew to go our separate ways. Jan and Darren were going to the airport together to catch their separate flights, returning one of the support cars in the process. There were more tears as we said goodbye. Jan urged me not to be too hard on myself.

"I've been amazed by your pain threshold," she told me. "It is beyond anything I have ever seen before. You put in a relentless effort, especially when it became clear your knee was causing you great discomfort. You still battled on." She continued: "I know you didn't achieve what we set out to do, but you still achieved an incredible performance of running over two thousand miles across America. I feel lucky to have been part of the team helping you do it. It certainly was a life experience I will never forget and I have made lifelong friends as a result."

She gave Tim a hug too and told him: "I'm glad Mimi has got you here to support her."

The dispersal of the crew in an RV park was a disappointing finish to what had been a great adventure, and certainly not the ending I had wanted. I felt everything had been rushed since I made the decision to stop. It would have been lovely if we could have all sat down together and enjoyed one last farewell meal before we split up. We could have chatted about things that had happened and shared some of the funny stories and experiences together. I was struggling to process what was happening and talking might have helped. One minute we were all together working towards one goal as a team, the next we were heading off in different directions. I know Tim felt the same way.

"It is a pity that the crew broke up so quickly," he said to me later when we got to our hotel. "It has left a bit of an empty hole. A good dinner and a drink or two with a moment to go over the many memories – good and painful – would have been a more fitting end."

He wanted this for me but also for himself, as a chance to say goodbye properly to everyone. I understood that the crew were exhausted and just wanted to go home though. Plus I wouldn't have been the greatest company as I was so disappointed in myself, and there was nothing they could have said to help.

* * *

I wasn't ready to go home yet: I wanted to hide away from the world in order to come to terms with what had happened and grieve the loss of the world record, and potentially my ultrarunning career. Physically and mentally I wasn't in a good place. I had contacted Becky to ask if she could arrange a hotel in New York for Tim and me as I simply didn't have the energy to do the research myself. Before going to the hotel, we returned the RV to a pre-arranged drop-off point where we were faced with a large bill for the damage Tim had done to the awning. We then travelled in the other support car to the hotel, where we had arranged for VW America to pick it up from the car park.

Tim and I rearranged our original flights home, bringing them forward but still allowing us to spend time in New York. I wouldn't actually be able to enjoy this time sightseeing in The Big Apple though, as I was still in so much pain. I could hardly walk. When we did leave the confines of our hotel room, poor Tim had to put up with me walking incredibly slowly – so slowly in fact that I had to laugh at myself on occasion: I must have looked as though I was a hundred years old. Tim loves to look around art galleries so he was keen to visit New York's famous Metropolitan Museum of Art. It took all my energy just to get there, so once inside the building, I sat down and waited an hour or so while Tim enjoyed seeing the exhibits.

I knew eating was an essential part of my recovery so for the first time in my life, I indulged in a large pretzel from a street vendor covered in chocolate. Boy, it tasted good. During the run I was lucky to be incredibly well fed by the crew. I can't believe how many delicious meals they cooked for me with the few ingredients they had. But even after eating huge quantities every day, I had still lost a lot of weight because of all the miles I had been doing. I would need to keep eating a lot to put some pounds back on. It wasn't just my weight that had suffered from all the calories I had been burning. I noticed when in New York that my hair looked much thinner than usual and my nails were weaker. About three weeks into the run, I had found that if I brushed my hair or washed it, I was losing many more strands than usual. I thought it was odd at the time, but I didn't dwell on it as I had more important things to worry about. When I returned home, my hairdresser commented on how much thinner my hair was and that I only just had new growth coming through. It seems that during and immediately after the world record attempt, my body diverted energy to where it was most needed – repairing my muscles, etc. – at the expense of strong hair and nail growth.

Although I wasn't in the right frame of mind to see anyone, I was absolutely overwhelmed with emotion when my former crew members and friends Becky, Paul and their two children came all the way from the UK to see me – that's true friendship. From the airport they went directly to their hotel, deposited their luggage then headed over to our hotel. My heart leapt for joy when we heard their knock on the door. Tim opened it and in rushed Becky who came straight over to the side of the bed I was sitting on and gave me the biggest hug for what seemed like ages. We both cried. We didn't need to say anything. I knew she understood exactly how I was feeling and that this hug from a best friend was exactly what I needed.

"I can't believe you are all here!" I exclaimed when we had regained our composure.

"We always intended to come for a family holiday," Becky said. "I was planning to be waiting for you along the last few miles of your route so I could leap out and surprise you and run with you to the steps of City Hall."

This made me cry all over again. I would have loved that. It would have been so special to have started and finished the run with Becky by my side.

"My heart broke when we got your text message to say you had to stop," Becky continued. "I knew I had to come and give you a hug. I knew you would need me more now than if you had succeeded and nothing would have kept me away."

We spent hours chatting about what had happened, and they kept reassuring me I hadn't failed. Their support enabled me to start the long journey of beginning to feel better about myself. That evening we went out for a celebratory meal. Even though I didn't feel like celebrating, it was marvellous to be in their company and I was so grateful they had made the effort to come out. The following day we did an open-top bus ride around New York, which was a much easier way for me to see the sights.

I knew people who had been following my journey and sponsored me deserved to know what had happened. But I felt so ashamed, I didn't want to talk about it and couldn't find the words to post anything online. Jenny had put a lovely statement on my website for me when we returned from the hospital, informing people why I had stopped, and I had been sent many supportive messages in response. Then Martin Yelling and Tom Williams contacted me and asked if

I would be willing to talk to them for their latest *Marathon Talk* podcast. It was the last thing I wanted to do as it was still so raw; I knew I wouldn't be able to speak without blubbing. But Tim said I shouldn't worry about being emotional as it showed how much I cared. Talking to them now would give a true reflection of how I felt. The show and its listeners have always supported me. I had spoken about my run and what I hoped to achieve to Martin on the show before I had left so I felt I owed it to them to explain what had happened. I wanted people to know I didn't give up; my body gave up on me.

When Tom called me in my hotel room, it was an emotional chat as I had expected. I tried my best to be upbeat, but I was fighting back tears for the whole conversation and struggling to contain my emotions. It was so hard to put into words how I felt – devastated and gutted didn't even cut it. My emotions went way beyond that; it was almost like a grieving process. Tom was great about making me feel better and helped me to see the positives from my journey.

"If this had been a challenge to run 2,215 miles across America in a phenomenal time, you would have achieved it with bells on," he told me.

It was lovely to recall the things I had enjoyed from the trip – the people I had met, the places I had seen, the generosity I experienced. People had gone out of their way to give me and the crew food and drinks, as well as handing over cash for the charities I was running for. Many others had generously donated online. I could take solace from the fact I had raised £7,706.84 for two very worthwhile causes. I knew it wasn't all negative; there were many reasons why I should have been proud of myself, but at that moment in time I was struggling to accept it. All I could see was the fact that I had failed.

To rub salt into my wounds, while I was in New York, Sandra made it to City Hall, setting a new female world record in the process. She had completed her journey in 54 days, 16 hours, and 24 minutes. One part of me felt happy for her. I knew how hard she would have worked for it and how much she deserved it for running so far every day for nearly eight weeks. I sent her a message of congratulations as soon as I could, and I meant every word. She had achieved something phenomenal and I respect and admire her for it. But another part of me felt sad and sorry that she had achieved something I couldn't. I'll admit I felt jealous. I wanted it to be me who had set a new world record. I felt awful for feeling that way.

When the day of our flight arrived, it was tough to be going home.

"What do I do now?" I asked Tim.

"Go back to normal, Mimi," he replied.

Back to reality and back to doing my own cooking, cleaning and laundry. I had become so used to everything being done for me, including the laying out of my kit the night before for me to put on the following morning, it was going to be a bit of a shock suddenly having to do everything myself! I was also slightly anxious about going home as I knew I would feel directionless. The record attempt had been my focus for so long and now it was over. I hadn't planned any other running events to look forward to as all I could think about in the build-up to America was America – there was no room to think about anything else. Someone said to me it must feel like when a celebrity gets kicked off *Strictly Come Dancing* and they wonder what to do with themselves now they no longer have dance practice every day and a live routine to perform on Saturday night. I felt lost and bereft, and, of course, the one thing that would make me feel better – running – I couldn't do.

I felt as though I was falling into a black hole of sadness. This kind of "post-marathon blues" is common for runners when a target race is over. You spend so many months working towards it and putting so much effort into training and the event itself, then suddenly it is all over. Afterwards, it feels as though you are utterly deflated; you feel completely flat as a pancake. I had felt this way after major challenges I had done before, but at least with the successful ones I also had the elation and satisfaction of knowing I had achieved what I set out to do. After America, on top of the emotions of feeling lost and flat, I also felt that I was a complete and utter failure. Many people said to me: "Mimi, you ran 2,215 miles in 40 days, how many other people ever do that? That isn't failure, that is a fantastic achievement." And yes, I did think it was amazing, but it wasn't what I set out to do. I set out to finish in New York on the steps of City Hall. That was my image, that was my vision. And I didn't. I finished in the hospital looking at an MRI scan.

Mentally I wasn't prepared for failure. Of course, I wasn't naive enough to think it couldn't happen, but it was always something I had pushed to the back of my mind in the build-up to, and during, the world record attempt. I had to do this because you need to believe in yourself completely in order to take on a challenge like this. Even when I had been in a lot of pain with sore legs and aching muscles in those last few weeks of the run, it never occurred to me to stop. I didn't contemplate that I wouldn't get to New York. My mindset had always been that I would get there no matter how much agony I was in. When I was going for that MRI scan, I was still 100 per cent certain that I was going to get to that finish line in New York. I couldn't have tried harder to get there.

I hadn't dwelled on failure before it happened because I felt that thinking about it would have been counterproductive. Fear of failure can stop people ever trying to achieve their dreams. I have never minded failing and I have failed in races and challenges in the past. It is a risk you have to take if you want to achieve something phenomenal. I always try to turn a failure (negative) into a positive; you can always learn from your mistakes. While I knew all this, I was still totally mentally unprepared for how to deal with failure after America. Perhaps it hit me so hard because it had been on such a large scale. It was a challenge I had been working towards for years, not just months. The preparation, planning and financial investment had been colossal.

On other occasions when I had failed, I had been able to look at why I hadn't finished, learn, and go back and have another go. For example, the first time I tried to run the double at the famous Spartathlon Ultra in 2013, I was unable to finish the race because I didn't eat enough and (I discovered later) I had a virus. I regrouped and returned in 2015. Having learned from my mistakes, I completed the 153-mile (246-km) race in Greece alongside the other competitors, then turned around to run back to the start on my own – a total of 306 miles (492 km). But I knew there would be no chance to re-run America. It was a once-in-a-lifetime challenge. Not only would it be too difficult and too expensive to plan again, there was the fact I might not even be able to run again, and certainly not long distances.

Were there lessons I could learn from the run across America? I didn't think so. Physically I couldn't have been more prepared. I had done all the training and all the rehab for my knee. I had found a route I was happy with. We did have to make some tweaks to it along the way, but because we had done the drive-through recce the year before, we avoided issues that would have caused major delays, so I have no regrets there. I never tried to do more mileage than I had planned unless it couldn't be avoided, which was sensible, although I did have days where I was forced to do less. Even with Sandra running a different route at the same time, I stuck to my plan. I wouldn't have changed the crew as they were all fantastic and worked incredibly hard. I ate enough to help me fuel and recover each day so I couldn't change anything there.

My knee was obviously a factor and some people may have thought it wasn't wise to try to go for the record a year after I had surgery for a torn meniscus. But I trusted my knee. I had done everything I could to rehabilitate it and make it strong again. My surgeon and all the other experts knew what I was doing and didn't think it was impossible. I had already had to delay the challenge twice, so I didn't want to delay it again. I don't think more time after the operation would have made any difference because I had done everything I could to recover. I never thought my knee would be my downfall. Even when I was starting to feel pain, I didn't think it was in my knee joint. I do wonder if wearing a knee brace earlier might have helped. But I still don't think it would have been enough to allow me to run another 600 miles (966 km) in time to achieve what I wanted, so there isn't much point looking back and wishing I had done things differently.

Given the choice I faced when I saw the results of the MRI scan, one thing I don't regret is stopping. I regret that it came to that, but I don't regret the decision not to continue in those circumstances. I think I would have been setting a very bad example if I had carried on running when I knew the state my body was in and how much was at stake. There are some injuries and niggles you can run through, and levels of pain you can tolerate. But there are other injuries when you have to admit that it is not possible and not worth running through them. I knew I couldn't keep on running just because I wanted to go and get a record. I would have been sending out a terrible message to other runners if I had done so. Sometimes you have to show people that actually it is not always worth it. With injuries we all get frustrated, we get angry because it means we have to pull out of races or can't do our planned training. But I have learned your overall health is much more important than a PB or a world record, or whatever it may be that you are trying to achieve at that moment.

* * *

Over time, after relaxing at home with my family and talking to friends and fellow ultrarunners, I did start to feel better about myself and what had happened. Gradually I was able to pull myself out of the black hole I had descended into. Stephen Hawking once said: "If you feel you are in a black hole, don't give up. There is a way out." He was right. I hadn't run across the whole of America and I hadn't set a new world record. But I had tried my hardest. I had run 2,215.24 miles (3,565.08 km) in 40 days. The final

0.24 miles is very important to me as I worked incredibly hard to cover it! I made it three quarters of the way across the third largest continent in the world. I had an amazing adventure with unforgettable experiences, met some fascinating people, and raised thousands for two wonderful charities. That isn't failure. That is something to be very proud of.

PART TWO:

OPENING NEW DOORS

CHAPTER SIX

DETERMINED TO RUN AGAIN

When I got back from America, I felt like there was a big void in my life. I missed running much more than I could have imagined. It had been such a massive part of who I was for the past two decades and now it had been taken away from me. I had become well known in the running community but I didn't know where I fitted into it any more. I felt completely lost. Could I even still call myself a runner now I wasn't able to run?

I watched Andy Murray's documentary, *Resurfacing*, and his experience really hit a nerve with me and reflected my own journey. I'm not comparing myself to his talent or achievements, but I could totally relate to how he felt when he faced having to give up the sport he loved because of a hip injury. Tennis is his passion, just like running is mine. He couldn't imagine his life without it and felt frustrated and upset that it could be taken away from him before he was ready to retire because one part of his body couldn't handle it. However, he didn't give up or accept it when he was warned he may never be able to play top-class tennis again. He researched his options, ended up having surgery and then did all the rehab he could to come back strong. In 2019, he won the doubles at Queens looking very much like his old self. I wasn't going to give up on the sport I loved either. I would explore all avenues to see if I could run again. I could accept that I may never be able to run long distances in the future, but I really struggled with the fact that I may never be able to run at all. Just to be able to run one kilometre would be better than nothing.

I turned to my friend Brett Rocos for advice. I had first met him while racing in the Jungle Ultra in Peru when his team, Exile Medics, were looking after the participants. He recommended I see an orthopaedic surgeon at Southmead Hospital in Bristol who specializes in knee surgery, as well as cartilage and ligament surgery for sportsmen and sportswomen. Bristol wasn't far from where my sister lived, so I stayed the night with her and she came with me to the appointment at the end of November 2017. Brett had already sent the MRI scan I had done in America, and I was hoping the surgeon would be able to come up with a miracle cure for my knee so I would be able to run again, ideally long distances. I was glad Jacqui was with me as it was an emotional experience. He explained everything extremely well and honestly, but it wasn't what I had hoped to hear. The reality of my situation was hard for me to listen to. He said it would be possible for me to run again, but only short distances. My ultrarunning days were over. No more multi-stage events, no more coast-to-coast world record attempts, no more competitive long-distance races. Even though in my heart of hearts I had known this would be the case, it was a blow to have it confirmed and I struggled to hold back the tears.

"You don't have to give up sport altogether," he told me. "You could do long-distance cycling and swimming."

Although I did later take up both sports, at the time it was not what I wanted to hear. I didn't want to do anything else. I wanted to run.

"Are there any options that would enable me to run further again?" I asked.

There were two surgical procedures he said were possibilities, but he didn't recommend either of them for me at the age I was at the time (the majority of knee replacements in the UK are carried out on 60–80 year olds and I was then 55).

"It is best to hang on to your joints as long as possible," he told me. "Both these options involve major surgery and unless you are in constant pain with your knee, I wouldn't advise it yet."

The first option was to have a half knee replacement. This involves just replacing one side of the knee. It involves a shorter hospital and recovery time than a full replacement, but doesn't last as long. The artificial joint would need redoing within ten years. This didn't sound like an appealing option to me. It meant having two operations within ten years – with all the rest, rehab and recovery that goes with it – plus the associated risks that come with any surgery. There was no guarantee I would be able to run further once I had recovered from the operation, and I was likely to wear it out faster if I did try to run too much.

The second option was to have an osteotomy. This involves having surgery where the bones are cut and reshaped. In the case of the knee joint, the tibia or femur may be cut to take pressure off the part of the knee joint which is damaged. The joint is held back together using metal plates and screws. It is a major procedure – and, again, came with no guarantee that I would then be able to run further than a half marathon afterwards. It would mean having a long period where I wouldn't be able to do much at all while I recovered. Again, this didn't sound like something I wanted to put myself through. I had done quite bit of reading and talking to people who had similar operations and I agreed with the surgeon, I would rather hold on to my body parts for as long as possible. Having surgery would mean I would be laid up for many more months and I would then only be able to do minimal exercise as I recovered.

I went home with a heavy heart. There was nothing I could do now except keep resting my knee and then hope that in a few months' time, I would be able to do the odd, short run again. It was a tough pill to swallow – and I wasn't ready to accept it yet. The following February, I arranged to see another knee specialist, who had been recommended to me by a number of other sportspeople he had helped, for a second opinion. I went to see him at his practice in Maidstone and hoped he might have some alternative options for me. His advice was exactly the same as I had been given before. He said I could run again but he thought a half marathon would be the maximum distance I could reach without risking further long-term damage. He also recommended I avoid any surgery for as long as I could, and instead do long-distance cycling if I wanted to take part in endurance events. I was gutted to hear the same thing again, but the fact these two experts both agreed made me realize there wasn't going to be a magical cure for me to be able to run ultras again. I had to look at the positives. These two surgeons had both recognized how important running is to me. They hadn't told me never to do it again, as some others might have done after seeing my MRI scan. But they had told me I had to be realistic and sensible. I wasn't going to be able to run far in the future, but I was going to be able to run a little. That was something positive.

I put my time and energy into learning more about cycling and swimming until I was strong enough to attempt running again. When I first got back from America, I struggled to move at all without pain in my knee. By the following March, I could cycle and swim, and I was able to do longer dog walks and easy cross training/walking on the treadmill in the gym without feeling any knee pain. By the middle of April, I had also regained the weight I had lost so my osteopath said I could try a run outside. This was the moment I had been longing for.

I drove to a forest not far from my house where I love to run and started walking to warm up. I was wearing a knee brace, as recommended by my osteopath, to give my knee some extra support. The plan was to walk for a few minutes and then break into a run. I was allowed to run up to one kilometre (0.6 miles) – as long as I was pain free. Despite being desperate to run for months, after walking for 15 minutes, I just couldn't pluck up the courage to try and run. I just kept walking and worrying. I was terrified in case my knee wouldn't hold up. What if the pain was still there after all these months? What if that meant I would never be able to run ever again? I realized I wouldn't know until I tried, so I took a deep breath and broke into a run. I started out with a gentle jog and was delighted everything felt good. I gradually picked up the pace and was overjoyed to be bounding along feeling no pain at all in my knee. I can't tell you how good that felt. The relief was overwhelming – and I burst into tears. I ran for a kilometre and then did the sensible thing and stopped as I had been advised. It might have only been a kilometre, but I was ecstatic to have been able to do it. If that was all I was ever able to do in the future, it was better than nothing.

After that, my joy at being able to run at all was slightly tempered with frustration because I couldn't simply run, I had to run-walk. The effort it took to do this felt extremely hard compared to how it had been when I was fitter. I was able to walk-run no more than twice a week up to 2 miles (3.2 km), till eventually I could run 3 miles (4.8 km) continuously – this seemed to take forever! If I did more than that, my knee would hurt, so there were weeks when I only did one run as I didn't want to overdo it. It felt as though I was back to where I was when I very first took up running. I couldn't believe that I used to be able to run hundreds of miles and do back-to-back marathons over multiple days. Now just doing 3 miles was a struggle. I had to keep reminding myself that I was fortunate to be able to run at all. Putting my trainers on and hitting the trails is my happy place and I was lucky it was still an option.

In October 2018, I arranged to see Shane Benzie in Goring-on-Thames, Berkshire, to have my running technique analysed. Shane is the founder of Running Reborn and has studied and researched running movement on six continents, coaching many people to improve their performance by tweaking their style. I couldn't think of a more qualified person to advise me. You may wonder why I wanted to improve my own technique given my days of running long distances and speedy PBs were over. The answer is I still want to be able to run, whatever the distance. Changing my technique could take some pressure off my bad knee, which could delay – or even better avoid – having knee surgery in the future. I had previously had my running gait analysed before going to America, but I wanted to do it again as my stride had changed as a result of my knee injury. It was a very different type of gait analysis too; Shane films his clients running outside, rather than on a treadmill, as you can run differently on the machines.

To analyse how I ran, Shane put sensors on both my legs and then, after a warm-up run around a field, he filmed me running away from and then towards him. I tried to run as naturally as possible which wasn't easy as I felt so self-conscious about being filmed and analysed. Watching the footage, I was shocked to see how much I was heel striking on my right leg. It looked as though I just threw my leg forward with no control, sending two and a half times my body weight up through my knee. My left leg landed in the right place, with a slight bend in the knee and more spring in the take-off. After discussing the problem areas with me, Shane then had me back running outside. This time, I had to try to stand taller and make an effort to land my right foot on the whole foot, rather than the heel. To be honest, I felt ridiculous – rather like a prancing pony – but my body certainly felt much springier. My feet were off the ground for longer and my right knee wasn't under as much pressure compared to my usual running form. Shane said this new movement would "dissipate the impact around the body and turn it into elastic energy".

Shane advised me to practise this new running style on every run. If I felt my new form go, I should stop, regroup and start again. In time, it would begin to feel much more natural and I would run this way without having to think about it. Shane told me: "Your movement is heavily influenced by your perception of it: change your perception and you change your movement." Once I had got the hang of it, he said I should arrange to go back and see him again to improve my form further. I definitely recommend getting this kind of advice if you want to improve and/or avoid injury. It is worth doing even if you have been running for twenty-odd years like me. I found it extremely beneficial and I am sure it will help protect my knee. If it helps me to keep running it is well worth it in my opinion.

CHAPTER SEVEN

PEDALLING BACK TO HAPPINESS

By the middle of December 2017, nearly two months after my return from America and before I was able to try running again, I was itching to exercise. I thoroughly enjoyed being able to walk my dog, as I find being in the fresh air really improves my mental health. But I missed being able to do other forms of exercise outside. After seeing the surgeon in Bristol, I kept thinking about his recommendation to take up long-distance cycling.

As I had been resting my knee and had regained some weight, I was given permission by my osteopath to use a static bike at the gym so long it was set on zero resistance. I could also do some gentle upper-body exercises using light weights.

After a couple of weeks using the static bike, my osteopath said I could try a bike ride in the great outdoors. I had bought a hybrid bike I call Marv (I like to give my bikes names) just before my knee operation in 2016 to use while

I was recovering and unable to run. At that time, it was also important for me to be able to get outside and exercise to get the endorphins pumping and just to feel more exhilarated and alive. I wasn't allowed to run outside for months after the surgery, so cycling was the next best thing. Back then, I would pedal around the country lanes near our house for around 15–30 miles (24–48 km). Tim would sometimes join me for shorter rides.

Although I have dabbled in cycling all my life, and I have been able to ride a bike from an early age, I would certainly have never described myself as a cyclist. While I love the fact that getting on a bike can get me out and about to exercise, it doesn't give me the same joy as running. It comes with a lot of extra worries for me – the terror of being hit by a car when cycling along roads and the fear of going into a pothole that could possibly propel me over the handlebars, resulting in a nasty injury. A situation similar to the latter is actually one of my first memories of riding a bike. I often cycled as a child but on one occasion when I was about eight years old, I remember cycling down a steep hill, losing control of the bike and going headlong into a sand box. I flew off my bike, went over a fence and crashed into a garden with a large dog in it: not a pleasant experience as the dog wasn't particularly friendly! Although it didn't put me off cycling, it made me feel less in control of my bike than I had felt before. From then on, I often didn't feel quite as safe when in the saddle.

Years later, while living in London in my twenties and working as a PA, I started cycling again as it was the easiest way to get to the office. It wasn't something I was doing for pleasure or exercise but simply a mode of transport and my best method of commuting. However, central London can be a dangerous place for a cyclist, and I was devastated one day to be told that a friend of mine had been killed in an accident when she had been cycling along Fulham Palace Road. It was a total shock, especially as I had only spoken to her a few days before to arrange a get-together with our group of friends. To receive this awful news was heartbreaking. I simply couldn't face cycling home at the end of the day, or in fact for a very long time afterwards. I started taking the Tube to work instead. My bike remained at the office for a long time. Eventually I had to get Tim to drive over and pick it up.

It wasn't until 1999 that I plucked up the courage to cycle again by agreeing to take part in the BallBuster Duathlon. By then I was a stay-at-home mother of three who had started going to the gym regularly for some "me time". It was there I made two wonderful friends – Maxine Ward and Louise Clamp – whose enthusiasm for exercise and love of a challenge had helped me get into running and sign up for events I never thought I could do. The duathlon was one of them. It is renowned for being particularly tough as the course takes in the very steep Box Hill in Surrey. By then, I had run my first half marathon so I felt I would be able to cope with the 8-mile (12.9-km) run and 24-mile (38.6-km) bike ride, followed by another 8-mile (12.9-km) run. After agreeing to take part, I realized I no longer owned a bike, so I thought I had better buy one! I bought a rather unattractive yellow road bike for £350. Knowing nothing about bikes, I had no idea whether it was a particularly good one. I was guided by what the bike shop assistant recommended, and more importantly, what was within my budget.

During the race, I felt physically strong, but I didn't enjoy the cycling section as much as the runs. I felt apprehensive on the downhills and found my bike to be really uncomfortable. Although it was hard work, I was determined to finish. Not only for personal pride but to prove wrong a marshal who had been less than encouraging as I was racking up my bike before the race. He asked me if I was part of a relay team. When I replied with a smile that I was taking part as an individual, he looked me up and down and said: "Very few women finish this event." No good luck or enjoy yourself, it seemed he simply didn't think women were capable of completing such a tough race. That really put the fire in my belly, and I knew I would finish no matter what. Many women finished that day, and many more have done it since, and faster than a lot of men. Over the years, women have shown over and over again that we are capable of anything we put our minds to.

Although I was proud to now call myself a duathlete, it wasn't something I was keen to do again in a hurry. The bike had really put me off cycling as it was so uncomfortable. It left me with some quite painful saddle sores afterwards – as all cyclists will know, chafing is very unpleasant! The bike went straight into the garage as soon as I got home, where it stayed for many years until I sold it. Running had now become the love of my life and after signing up for the Marathon des Sables with Max and Louise, training for that became my full focus. Since then, cycling had been something I only dabbled in as a last resort when I wasn't able to run.

At the end of December 2017 when my osteopath gave me permission to start cycling outside, he said I could go twice a week initially. I had to take things slowly and stop if I felt any pain in my knee. I was still recovering from America, so I wasn't back to full form in terms of energy, so twice a week was plenty to begin with. This was a huge step forward, making me feel a lot more positive.

Thankfully, once I started pedalling, my knee felt fine and it was wonderful to be out in the fresh air. It just didn't give me the same buzz as running though, and I would feel a pang of jealousy whenever I cycled past a runner. I wished I could have been pounding the pavements in my trainers like they were, instead of riding my bike. I knew it was such a negative way to think and that I would be better off focusing on, and appreciating, what my body could do, rather than what it couldn't. But I couldn't help it. I missed my running so much. I missed heading up to the forest or meeting up with friends for a run. I missed the motivation of having an event to train for. I needed to talk to someone who had been in a similar situation to me, so I turned to my friend Mark Cockbain.

Mark had been an incredible ultrarunner, taking on some of the toughest races in the world, but unfortunately his running career came to an end when his knees started causing him issues. I knew he would understand what I was going through and that he would be honest with me about what to expect in the future. He recommended I enter a cycling race so that I had something to aim for and work towards, as this was something I was definitely missing since returning from America.

"But I know nothing about cycling races!" I told him.

Knowing I like a challenge, he suggested I enter the Deloitte Ride Across Britain (RAB). I had a look at their website and discovered it is a 980-mile (1,577 km) cycling event from Land's End to John o'Groats staged over nine days. It's a ride and an experience rather than race so there was no pressure to be competitive. But I immediately dismissed the idea as I thought there was no way I could cycle that far. It involved covering 100 miles (161 km) or more a day. Plus, it was very expensive to enter as it is a fully supported ride, which means entrants are provided with hot food, mechanical and medical support, tented accommodation, and have massages and sports nutrition advice available to them the whole way. I would then have additional travel expenses, namely getting to the start at Land's End and getting home from John o'Groats. I would also have to pay to get my bike delivered to the race start and home again afterwards. Oh, and there was the fact I didn't own a suitable road bike to do the ride on!

It's not for me, I thought, logging off the website. However, for days afterwards I kept thinking about it. I knew I needed something to help me feel more positive again and get me out of the dark hole I found myself descending into. Coincidentally, 2018 would be the ten-year anniversary of my Guinness World Record run from John o'Groats to Land's End, so I reasoned it would be an apt way to celebrate. Then I would have run AND cycled the length of Great Britain. I found myself looking at the website again and had to admit, the ride sounded as though it would be a wonderful adventure, just what I was looking for.

"From the rolling hills of Cornwall to the vast, sweeping landscapes of Scotland, you will explore the best cycling Britain has to offer, passing iconic locations such as St Michaels Mount, Cheddar Gorge, The Severn Bridge, Forth Bridge and The Lecht Pass," the course description read. I couldn't resist signing up.

When I told Tim, he wasn't at all surprised. "Typical!" he said with a smile on his face. He was shocked when I told him how much it was going to cost, but he was also pleased I was excited about something for the first time since coming back from America. I think he had been waiting for me to announce which crazy challenge I was going to do next. This was certainly going to be a big ask for me; the furthest I had ever cycled before signing up was around 30 miles (48 km). I knew nothing about what was involved to prepare for a bike ride of this duration. But this didn't phase me, as I had known nothing about long-distance running when I had first taken it up, and I had managed to learn and excel. Hopefully cycling would be the same. The event wasn't until September, so I had plenty of time to get ready.

My hybrid bike Marv would be unsuitable for a ride of this duration as it is quite heavy. What I needed was a road bike. In the January, I contacted a friend who owns a bike shop in Scotland asking for advice as to which was the best to get on my budget. Ideally, I wanted it to be pink! Unfortunately, there wasn't anything in this colour unless I was prepared to pay a vast amount of money (which I didn't have). I wasn't looking for anything too fancy; so long as it could get me from one end of the country to the other with relative ease I was happy. He recommended the Specialized Dolce, a female-specific bike in my price range. I ordered it online and went to a bike shop in Maidstone to pick it up. It was an orangey red colour so if I squinted it became pink! I decided to call her Mavis. To make up for the lack of pink on the frame, I ensured my helmet and as much of my kit as possible were pink instead.

Over the next few months, I started to get several niggles in my lower back and neck, making riding extremely uncomfortable. Local cycling friends highly recommended going to a bike shop in Tunbridge Wells where I could have a professional bike fit known as a "Retül". This bike fit would take about 3 hours as it was very thorough. They asked me about any injuries and my cycling history as well as taking various body measurements. They then placed LED markers on eight anatomical points of my body, which enabled the Retül Vantage Motion Capture system to track my movements as I pedalled. The data collected was used to make adjustments to my position on the bike.

A bike fit like this is well worth the time as it can make a big difference to your power, comfort and efficiency on the bike (even for an amateur like me!). The changes they made took the pressure off my back and knees, making cycling much more comfortable. It was a revelation and made a huge difference to how I felt when riding. I highly recommend anyone who rides a bike regularly has this kind of fitting as the smallest tweaks can make a massive difference. I probably would have enjoyed cycling a lot more in the past if I had been riding a bike that had been adjusted to fit me.

I gradually started increasing the time I spent out on Mavis and, to my surprise, the more I cycled, the more I began to enjoy it. I had absolutely no pain in my knee and my legs felt strong when I pedalled, even when going up tough hills. I actually found going up easier than going down, as downhills left me feeling completely out of control. Every time I went down a steep hill my hands would be firmly on the brakes as I didn't enjoy the feeling of going fast. Most people love it, but I worried about the potholes, or coming to a corner and not being able to make the turn. I had always been on two feet so two wheels would take a bit of getting used to.

The first few times I went out cycling, I was so scared about taking my left hand off the handlebars to indicate turning left, I only chose routes where I could make right turns! When I was only using one hand, Mavis would wobble all over the place making me feel extremely vulnerable, especially if there were vehicles coming towards me. After several rides everything became easier, until eventually I didn't even have to think about it. At this point, apart from the helmet and an old pair of cycling tights, all the clothes I wore when out riding was my running kit. Basically, I was a runner on a bike! Gradually over the next few months in the build-up to the RAB I bought myself some proper cycling kit and slowly began to look and feel a bit more like a cyclist.

As with my running, I would do most of my bike rides alone as I found it easier to fit everything in that way. A friend advised me it would be a good idea to try to meet up with other cyclists more often so I could get used to riding in a group ahead of the RAB. There are many benefits to cycling in a group. I could discover new routes, meet new people, and learn the safety aspects of cycling with others, such as where to position myself when a car is overtaking, and how to avoid getting too close to the wheel of the cyclist in front or beside you to avoid a nasty collision. I would also learn the various hand signals cyclists use to warn one another there is a pothole coming up, or an obstacle to cycle round. I knew very little about all this.

After a bit of searching online, I discovered a newly formed group in my area called Headcorn Wheelers. I made contact with them and after an initial chat over the phone, signed up for their next ride. I felt like the new girl at school when I first went to meet them, but everyone was very friendly and welcoming. I began riding with them every Sunday which added a fun and sociable element to my cycling. I loved gleaning lots of information from the other cyclists who had more experience (and admittedly more passion at the time!) for cycling than me. I started to become familiar with various parts of the bike – such as the hanger. Previously I thought this was something you put clothes on! And I learned how to fix a puncture, definitely an essential part of cycling. I'm hoping that as time goes on I will become faster at putting in a new inner tube!

One thing I struggled to get to grips with was clipless pedals (also known as clip-in pedals). They were the cause of a couple of meltdowns. For those who are as clueless about cycling as I was, these require special shoes with two- or three-bolt cleats in a specific pattern that clip into the pedals. One of the benefits of clipless pedals is that they help you go faster because you generate power both when you push down on the pedal, and when you pull up. Being clipped into your pedal also stops your foot from moving around, keeping it in a better position for more efficient riding. However, I absolutely hated them. My first pair of shoes were the ones worn by the majority of road cyclists with three-bolt cleats. They were a nightmare. Every time I wore them, I fell off Mavis as I wasn't able to unclip my shoe from the pedal to dismount so I would topple over onto my side. They were also really uncomfortable to walk around in when not on the bike because the cleats stick out from the base of the shoe. I have heard people say it looks as though you are walking like a penguin! I reverted to good old-fashioned flat pedals and trainers and felt much better for it.

Another string to my cycling bow was getting a turbo trainer. This is a gadget that transforms a pedal bike into a static bike so you can exercise in the comfort of your own home. It is a great training aid on days when it is too wet or icy to go outside. Much like treadmill running, it can get a little boring, so I help pass the time by watching films and listening to podcasts and music. A few people recommended a cycling app called Zwift, so I decided to try it. It allows you to ride routes around the world virtually and interact with other cyclists. I was immediately hooked as it made me feel part of the cycling community and added variety to my training when pedalling away inside on my own.

As the date of the RAB drew closer, I started increasing my rides to build up my endurance. I was already doing tempo and threshold sessions on my turbo to increase my stamina, but now I also needed to up the mileage on my longer rides outside. Having looked at the profile of the race I knew there were going to be some massive hills on the route, both steep uphills and downhills. The ascents would include the Cheddar Gorge and Shap Fell in England, and Glenshee and Lecht Hill in Scotland. The highest ascent we would climb was 8,232 ft (2,509 m).

During my training I tried to cycle as many hilly routes as I could. Stupidly, I didn't think about doing a hill rep session as I would have done in running (i.e. going up and down the same hill a number of times). From a confidence point of view, I wanted to get in at least one 100-mile (161 km) ride (realistically I should have done more) to practise eating and drinking, as well as testing out some of my kit. This is something I always did in the build-up to my running events to check everything was comfortable and didn't chafe. I decided to give clipless pedals another go, but this time went for SPD shoes and pedals which are favoured by mountain bikers. They have two-bolt cleats that are recessed into the base of the shoe, making walking easier. They revolutionized my cycling; I absolutely loved them.

I had the perfect opportunity to try my first 100-mile (161-km) ride in June when a local war hero who lived in my village turned 100. To celebrate, another local, Carl Adams, organized a 100-mile run doing loops of 10 miles around Smarden, Kent. He encouraged everyone to get involved in some way, whether that was running one loop of 10 miles, walking a loop as a family, or handing out water and food at the Smarden Sports Pavilion to the ultrarunners. It was a wonderful way to honour our local hero and his service to the country on Armed Forces' Day. As I couldn't run, I asked if I could cycle instead, and thankfully Carl agreed. This was going to be a huge learning curve for me as it was the furthest I had ever cycled. I practised eating and drinking on the bike, used my house (which was slightly off the route) as a checkpoint to top up my water and food, and practised unclipping my left foot each time I came to a junction, just in case I had to stop and put my foot down. Obviously, as I was on a bike, I completed the miles before the ultrarunners – who would be running for more than 24 hours. After finishing my century, I went to bed and got up very early the next morning to get back on my bike and go in search of the runners to give them support for the final few hours of their run. The camaraderie was wonderful, and I felt very honoured to have been part of such a great event, even though I couldn't run.

In the July before the RAB, my friend, Caroline Richards, agreed to ride coast to coast (or "sea to sea" as it is also known) across England with me. This is a 140-mile (225-km) route from Whitehaven, Cumbria, to Tynmouth, Tyne and Wear. It is one of the most popular long-distance cycle routes in the country and is usually ridden from west to east to make use of the prevailing winds. You can do it as part of an organized ride, but we decided we would do it on our own so there would be no pressure to reach checkpoints and we would save money on entry fees. There would be some huge hills to climb along the way as we would pass through the Lake District and North Pennines. The highest point we would reach would be over 1,998 ft (609 m). I was nervous about how I would fare on the steep inclines and sharp descents, but I knew it would be great training for the RAB.

It is traditional for cyclists to put their rear wheel into the Irish Sea in Whitehaven at the start of the ride (and their front wheel into the North Sea at Tynmouth at the end) so we decided to join in with this rite of passage before we set off. Trying to put our rear wheel in at the start was somewhat tricky though as the slipway down to the water was incredibly slippery and manoeuvring our bikes down the steep slope nearly ended up with both Caroline and myself going for a swim!

I had decided to ride on Marv, my hybrid bike, as he was better suited to some of the off-road sections we would be tackling. It did make cycling on the roads harder though as he is heavier than my road bike, Mavis. Cycling through the Lakes was fantastic with views of the hills all around. The uphill sections here were tough but I was never forced to get off and push. The Hartside Summit in Alston, Cumbria, to nearly 2,000 ft (610 m) above sea level, was particularly hard work. According to the guidebook I had bought, it wasn't "the hardest climb" so my pride meant getting off the bike to walk here definitely wasn't an option! It felt relentless but it wasn't the steepest hill we encountered so I simply had to keep pedalling. There used to be a cafe at the summit popular with cyclists and bikers travelling along the Hartside Pass. We would have loved to have taken a break there, but it burned down in 2018. It has since been rebuilt so perhaps I will have to go back one day for a well-earned coffee and cake.

A harder climb from Garrigill to Nenthead was awaiting us in the afternoon. According to the guidebook, this is the most brutal climb on the whole route. It is only 1.5 miles (2.4 km) long but it definitely felt longer, with the first section being very steep. This was one where I just had to grind it out to the top. The views across the Pennines when we reached the summit were worth all the hard work.

We didn't want to rush the trip, so we allowed three days to complete the ride. Despite getting lost on a couple of occasions, we completed the 140 miles in just under two and a half days. This gave us time to have a delicious lunch overlooking the sea when we finished before having to cycle to the station to catch our pre-booked train home to Kent. Having no pressure to finish as quickly as possible made for a much more relaxed and enjoyable journey. On the train home, I was tired, elated and proud to have finished my first long-distance cycling adventure. It had been a fantastic experience, especially doing it with a friend. Completing the journey without any hitches made me feel much more confident and excited about taking part in the RAB.

The remaining build-up to the RAB was both exciting and nerve-racking. As with any event, I tried to have everything organized well in advance. I decided to have Mavis sent on to Land's End ahead of me (which is what most people did), rather than have the issue of getting her to the start myself. Mavis was picked up from my house a week early so she would be ready and waiting for me when I got there. It felt strange packing her up and sending her off without me; I was becoming quite attached to this little machine!

The night before I was due to leave, I had my usual pre-race nerves. Except this time, rather than worrying about what could go wrong with me, as I did before a running event, I was concerned about my bike. I worried about silly things, such as how often should I oil the chain, and whether to check the tyre pressure at the end or beginning of each day. I even went onto YouTube to learn how to fix my chain should it break, although I'm not sure I would have felt totally competent doing it for real! I opted for tubeless tyres as a lot of people had said this was definitely the way to go, as it takes me ages to change an inner tube if I get a puncture and I didn't want to get left behind.

Running is so much easier! I thought as I tried to push my worries to one side so I could get a good night's sleep. I reassured myself that as with my running races, everything would fall into place once I started. Any situation that occurred I would try to deal with as best I could. If not, I was going to be surrounded by experienced cyclists and have the support of the RAB organizers and their mechanics along the course. If I had a problem I couldn't fix, I could be sure someone would be able to help me.

My good friends Becky and Paul, who crewed for me in America, live in Cornwall so I stayed with them the night before heading to the camp the following morning – a lovely, relaxed way to prepare for my first big cycling event. Becky drove me to Land's End in their van, bringing a large mattress in the back so she could sleep in it that night and wave me off the following morning. Having parked up, it was great to meet and chat to a few fellow cyclists, many of them were also doing the RAB for the first time. Becky and I were incredibly impressed by the very slick set-up of the event. I started to feel less nervous and more excited. There were around 800 participants, so it felt similar to a music festival with loads of activity everywhere and a huge campsite.

Although some people opted to stay in hotels, the majority would camp so there were rows and rows of tents set up in long lines. Everyone would be assigned their own individual tent. There were stalls for coffee and food in one area, and portable toilets, showers and changing rooms in another. Unlike at most music festivals though, these toilets were actually quite plush. They even had a tent with hair driers and straighteners – everything was provided.

The main marquee was something to behold. Inside was an area where participants could relax on giant beanbags. They had yoga mats for people to use, and a very long table at the back of the marquee with loads of charging points for devices such as mobile phones and navigation aids. In the middle there was a massive dining area with long trestle tables and chairs. To the side were tables with coffee and teas as well as other drinks. And then there was the food! The food was something else: I don't think I have ever seen so many delicious-looking meals and snacks under one roof. They catered for everyone, whatever their dietary requirements. It really was very impressive. This set-up would be replicated every night along the way; the organization was second to none.

It was also wonderful to be reunited with Carol and her film crew in Land's End. She wanted to do some more filming for the documentary as she felt covering my RAB adventure, and how I coped with the different challenge, would be a good end to the story. She also wanted to do a few more interviews with me about the run across America and how I had been since returning home. We all walked to the Land's End signpost for a few photos. I then did all the final checks ahead of the ride that would start at 7 a.m. the following morning, including attaching my number to Mavis, once I had located her racked up among all the other hundreds of bikes.

There seemed to be a lot of professional-looking cyclists around so I felt a little out of my depth. I reminded myself that I often thought this at the start of an ultra when other runners looked like "proper" runners and I would begin to compare myself unfavourably to them. I put that thought to one side and concentrated on the adventure ahead of me. Once my admin had been done, Becky and I went to Carol's accommodation where she filmed an interview with me. There were several occasions when I found answering her questions extremely emotional as they brought back many memories, good and bad. With the interview completed we headed back to camp for the compulsory 8 p.m. meeting to go over the safety measures for the event and the route for the following day.

With the meeting over, I headed to my tent and settled in for my first night under canvas. The tents were designed for two people but everyone had one to themselves so there was plenty of room to sleep as well as space for our luggage. I was more than happy for this to be my home for the duration of the journey. The atmosphere in the camp was very relaxed, and people were enjoying beers and sitting around chatting. I had decided I wouldn't drink alcohol throughout the ride as after a long day cycling, I knew I wouldn't really enjoy a glass of wine. It would most likely just give me an almighty headache as I would be dehydrated, and it was better to stay clear-headed.

We were set off in waves the next morning with about 20 riders starting at a time. In theory, the slower riders went first as we all had to be finished by 7 p.m., but many of the faster riders would also set off early. A few of them arrived at the next camp before it had been set up. I couldn't imagine cycling that fast, but it would also give them longer to recover.

I cycled with my friends Paul and Phil who I had done a couple of rides with prior to the RAB as we all live in Kent. It was great to have their company and certainly helped ease my nerves as we rode past the moors and up and down the many West Country hills. It was just as well we had fresh legs, as the first day was the hilliest day of the whole route with 8,232 ft (2,509 m) of ascent as we passed through Cornwall and into Devon to finish the day in Okehampton.

Passing through the same places I had gone through when running the JOGLE world record brought back so many memories. As I had run that north to south, by the time I had reached Devon and Cornwall I was really digging deep and in a lot of pain, so I hadn't been able to take in too much of my surroundings. It was nice to be on day one of my cycle ride going through a few familiar places feeling much fresher and able to enjoy the sights along the way, including St Michael's Mount. As I wasn't up against the clock like I had been in 2008, it was also wonderful to be able to stop and take pictures if I wanted to without having to worry about wasting time. To add to the day, Becky would pop up at various points along the route to wave at us which always brought a smile to my face.

The following day brought yet more hills as we skirted around the edge of Dartmoor and then up the Cheddar Gorge. I had been worried about this section because everyone had told me how difficult it was as the gradient was 16 per cent at one point. As with all the hills, I told myself I just had to keep my feet turning in endless circles and ignore my burning leg muscles; eventually I would reach the top. It turned out it was only the first part of the gorge climb that was really steep as we snaked up with the tall, grey rocks of the gorge on either side. It wasn't as bad as I had expected and, once the gradient levelled out, the remaining couple of kilometres were much easier, allowing me to enjoy the views and even chat to a few people as they overtook me.

As we got closer to the top, we had even better views of the striking moors and land below. But what goes up, must come down. As I still wasn't very confident on the descents, I didn't enjoy the next downhill section. It was then on to our final destination of the day, the beautiful Roman city of Bath. It would have been lovely to visit one of the famous Roman spas to recover in their healing waters, but I made do with a hot chocolate while putting my feet up on my bed. I had a real bed for this night as our accommodation was at Bath University rather than in tents.

From Bath, we headed over the Bristol Channel on the Severn Bridge. I was relieved there was a designated cycle lane so the passing traffic didn't feel too close when overtaking. Crossing this iconic bridge had given me a real boost when I had been running JOGLE as it had come at a time when I had been really struggling to keep going and worrying that the world record was slipping further out of reach. It felt much more relaxing this time to be crossing without any time pressure on me and with my legs feeling much fresher than they had ten years before.

The next section of the ride took us along the River Wye after a pit-stop at Chepstow Castle. I had been told this was one of the most beautiful sections of the ride and it really was. The route was constantly lined with cyclists stopping on quaint bridges and beside sweeping views of the river below to take photos. We often stopped to take in the beauty all around us too. *This is exactly why I want to have adventures like this*, I thought at one of our breaks as I looked out over the peaceful water and unspoilt countryside beyond. I felt lucky I was still able to reach places like this on my bike now I couldn't run through them in ultra-marathon events.

I found cycling day after day couldn't really be compared to running a multi-day event. Physically, I found it easier ticking off the miles on a bike as there wasn't the constant pounding on the body. The miles passed much more quickly too which made it easier mentally. Running 100 miles could take me anything from 17.5 to 30 hours but when cycling I could cover the ground in about 9 hours. Of course, cycling can have a huge toll on your body with the distances we were covering each day, but it helped that I wasn't pushing myself to my limits as I often did in an ultrarun. I wasn't racing; I was enjoying the experience. I found carrying essential kit on the bike was also much easier than running with a vest or rucksack. I had a saddle bag which had my waterproof and windproof jacket in, and two bottle cages for my water on the frame; much simpler.

Thankfully I didn't suffer from saddle soreness or feel too fatigued each day. I was having a ball, enjoying the scenery and meeting new people. Mentally and physically I was in a good place and found getting up each morning to cycle 100 miles or more wasn't an issue. I never felt negative or reluctant to ride. It definitely made a difference having good weather and virtually no rain. Once the sun came up, it made for very enjoyable cycling weather. I was told the year before they had been extremely unlucky as it had poured with rain from start to finish.

Each day we had three pit-stops where we could get food, replenish our water and rest if needed. These were approximately 30 miles (48 km) apart. Just like in an ultra race, the pit-stops (or checkpoints as we call them in ultra races) were always a good goal and something to look forward to. Another difference I noticed was that in an ultra race, you tend to get to a checkpoint, grab what you need – whether that is food or topping up your water bottles – and then get going again as soon as possible. The pit-stops in the RAB were much more laid back. Everyone seemed to be happy to take their time queuing for food, chatting, eating, drinking and just going with the flow before getting going again. Personally, I found this a little frustrating as once I was in the rhythm of cycling, I wanted to complete each stage as quickly as possible. I had to remind myself this wasn't a race, it was a journey, so there was no rush. The only requirement was for everyone to be finished each day by 7 p.m. I didn't notice anyone being competitive but I'm sure the speedy ones at the front were competing against one another, even though it wasn't an official race!

The route across England continued through Ludlow to Haydock and then up into the Lake District where we faced climbing the mighty Shap Fell, which is 1,397 ft (426 m) above sea level. As usual, my aim was to reach the top without falling off my bike. Rather than being short and steep, the climb was a long one at nearly 4 miles (6.4 km) but I was able to maintain a steady pace and keep going.

By day six we passed the border into Scotland which felt like a massive achievement. It also brought a change in temperature. Waking up after the first night in the grounds of Hopetoun House, on the outskirts of Edinburgh, it was absolutely freezing. I had to start the day with all my cycling kit on – long-sleeved base layer, my warmest cycling jersey, gilet, gloves and my waterproof jacket – and I was still chilly. Everyone said they couldn't feel their hands on the handlebars as they had gone numb from the cold. I knew my motherland would offer us some spectacular scenery to ride through and it didn't disappoint. I told myself the great views at the top of the steep hills I was struggling to ride up would make it all worth it. I noticed lots of people zigzagged up the very harsh inclines to make it easier. There were a few sections where the gradient was over 20 per cent. On some occasions, I would be working hard up a hill and start to overtake someone who I could tell was really struggling to find any power to keep pedalling forward. Sometimes, they would completely run out of puff and then just fall on their side. As I was struggling to keep going and stay upright myself, I wasn't able to stop and help but they would give a thumbs up to say they were OK.

Despite all my worrying in the build-up about my lack of experience and cycling endurance, I found there were others taking part who weren't as fit and hadn't trained as much as me. Not everyone completed the stage each day on their bike. Some people needed to get into the "death bus" as it was called, where they would be driven back to camp. For some, that would be the end of their journey; others would continue the following day. Some participants had only signed up to cycle through England, so they finished their rides when we reached Edinburgh. They were replaced by a large contingent of fresh-legged cyclists who had entered just the Scottish stages.

I quickly learned why these stages were so appealing. We went through some of the most beautiful countryside on single-track roads. The scenery really was breathtaking with many "WOW" moments as we passed magnificent hills and lochs sparkling in the sun. The weather remained clear and dry so there was no rain or mist to spoil the views. During my JOGLE World Record I had run down the A9 while in this area, a pretty scary road, so it was wonderful to be cycling towards John o'Groats through such glorious scenic backroads instead. I would never have believed in 2008 that a decade later I would be making my way back to John o'Groats, but this time on a bike.

It felt amazing after nine days of cycling and 980 miles to finally reach the coast. Crossing the finish line with Paul and Phil was incredibly special. We had spent the duration of the journey together, giving each other support when needed, space when required but always being there for one another. Carol was there to capture the moment. She told me she was stunned at how fresh I looked after cycling the length of the country.

"You look like you've just popped out for a pint of milk!" she exclaimed. "How do you feel?"

"Marvellous!" I replied.

I had set myself two goals at the start. The first was to finish, and the second was to cycle up all the hills and not get off to walk. I was delighted I had managed to achieve both. I felt as though I had finally closed a chapter of my life that hadn't been easy. I hadn't succeeded in America, but I had somehow picked myself up, discovered cycling, and completed another epic journey. I felt like my old self again. I had set myself a tough challenge and I had conquered it.

I had hoped to have my picture taken under the famous John o'Groats sign but there was a massive queue of other cyclists wanting to do the same thing, and I had to get Mavis to her transport and catch my bus to Inverness. In the end, we managed to find a spot where Carol could get the sign in the background of the shot. I beamed for the camera beside my bike with my medal proudly hung around my neck. I had now travelled the length of Great Britain on two feet and two wheels. Both had been slightly different routes and I experienced different levels of pain and euphoria – but both are major achievements that I am extremely proud of.

CHAPTER EIGHT

BATTLING MY UNDERWATER DEMONS

From a young age I have been terrified of water. It stemmed from my childhood and an incident with an abusive nanny who had been hired to look after my younger sister, Jacqui, and me. My parents had no idea what a monster she was. We were too frightened to tell them as this nanny from hell threatened to kill us if we did. She terrorized us for months when we were living in Norway, where my father had been posted as a Colonel in the British Army to work with NATO. It was due to her mental and physical abuse that I later developed the eating disorder that could have cost me my life.

I starved myself for years because of that woman (the only way I refer to her now). She was a cruel bully who constantly told me I was worthless and ugly and deserved the beatings and punishments she constantly inflicted on me. We were finally rid of her when my mother noticed bruises and scratches all over my body caused by the nanny pulling me down a flight of stairs by my legs. I found the courage to tell my mother the truth and we never saw that woman again. But while she was out of our lives, it wasn't so easy to banish her from my head. There were still times, decades later, when she would creep back into my mind and I would feel like the scared little girl at her mercy again. And those times were when I faced being in water.

My mother said it hadn't always been that way. She told me that I could "swim before I could walk", as I used to love paddling and splashing about in rivers, picking up pebbles from the riverbeds. The fear of water developed one day when I was seven years old, and I watched Jacqui, then five, nearly drown. The nanny had taken us for a walk along a river in Norway when it was iced over in the bitterly cold winter months. Jacqui and I had a ball with us which we had been happily playing with before the nanny seized it and kicked it across the ice.

"Well, go and get it back then!" she ordered my sister.

"I can't!" Jacqui replied. "What if I fall through the ice?"

"Don't make her do it," I pleaded.

The nanny wouldn't budge and insisted Jacqui walk over the thin ice to retrieve the ball. I could barely breathe as I watched a terrified Jacqui tentatively step onto the frozen river and attempt to walk slowly towards the ball, the ice creaking and cracking beneath her feet. Sure enough, she had only gone a few steps when – crack! – the ice gave way completely and Jacqui fell into the freezing water. She screamed in shock and flailed her arms in her desperate bid to stay afloat, causing more of the ice to break up around her and push her along the river as the current flowed. Watching it all unfold on the riverbank I felt utterly helpless.

"Do something!" I screamed at the nanny. "You have to help her, she might drown!"

With absolutely no sense of urgency, the nanny reached Jacqui's position and held her leg over the water so she could grab on to it to pull herself out of the water. I rushed to help drag my sister back onto the bank, hugging her to try and give her back some warmth as she was shivering and soaked through. The nanny offered no comfort and didn't show any concern. She just looked down on us and said: "Don't tell anyone about this, or next time, I'll push you both in the river and you won't get out again."

I would often have nightmares where I would relive the moment that I saw Jacqui falling into the river, crying out for help with her face full of fear. I couldn't forget how I felt totally helpless and powerless to save her from my position on the bank. That feeling of anxiety and fear of water has stayed with me ever since. It made me realize how deadly open water can be with its hidden strong currents and freezing temperatures. Sometimes even the strongest swimmer wouldn't have a chance of survival, let alone a swimming novice like me if I got into trouble. So rather than face my fears, I tried to forget them by avoiding water as much as possible.

When I returned from America though, going to my local leisure centre pool twice a week was recommended as a key element of my knee rehab. My osteopath said "water walking" would aid my recovery. This involves walking around in circles in the shallow end of the pool. Walking in water is harder than walking normally because it offers natural resistance that can help strengthen the muscles. As the water also gives buoyancy, it takes pressure off the joints. I looked ridiculous and I didn't enjoy being in the water, but I was prepared to do it if it would help re-strengthen my knee.

When I first started going, a lady came up to me and said she was worried about me when she first saw me walking to get into the pool as my movement was so pained and awkward. But once in the pool, she was relieved to see I could always move more easily and looked better every time she saw me.

"I was amazed when I first saw you were getting into the pool when you could barely walk," she told me. "I take my hat off to you, you never gave up."

As I was going to the pool at the same time twice a week, I soon got to know many of the other regular swimmers. I envied them breezing up and down doing lengths while I remained in the shallow end walking. I did know how to do breaststroke, but I would always swim with my head firmly above the water. I longed to be able to do front crawl but that had always been out of the question for me as it involved putting my head into the water, which I found terrifying.

The more I went to the pool, the more I felt it was such a shame I wasn't actually swimming and that a childhood fear was still dominating my life so much. It had affected many family holidays we had been on in the past and had meant I had never been able to fully relax and enjoy swimming with my children. I was always fearful when we were near water in case something happened to them. When I was in a swimming pool with my children, I always did my best to hide my fear as I didn't want to pass it on to them. They had no idea how I felt – they saw me doing breaststroke so thought everything was OK.

There were many occasions when my kids thought it was hilarious to try to dunk Mummy in the water. If they succeeded, I would flail around under the water, panic rising up inside me before breaking free to the surface with a gasp of relief. I would then dash to the side and grip on for dear life. Not only did it awaken the memories of Jacqui falling into the icy river, it also caused me to relive something else traumatic that once happened to me when we lived in Norway. We had swimming lessons once a week at school and during one of the lessons a boy held me under the water with his feet on my shoulders. I was terrified I was going to drown.

My children didn't know about any of this, but my initial reaction was to feel angry with them for bringing back these bad memories. I knew I had to resist the urge to give them a telling off as they didn't understand. They just thought we were playing a fun game. It would be amazing if I could overcome my fears so I could fully enjoy swimming with my grandchildren. I also wanted to be able to do some form of exercise if we went on a holiday where running or cycling wasn't an option.

My fear of water nearly prevented me completing the Jungle Ultra in 2012. This 146-mile (235-km) six-day staged race held in Peru involved approximately 57 river crossings on the longest day alone. Most of them were easy as the water was shallow enough to walk through but, in other places, there was such a strong current that ropes were stretched across the water for us to hold onto to cross without being swept away. The first time I reached a deep crossing, my heart rate went through the roof. My body began to shake and all I wanted to do was cry. The memory of Jacqui falling into the river in Norway and being swept along by the current was all I could think of.

How on earth am I going to get across? I thought.

Thankfully, a fellow runner called Kenny who I had talked to about my fear before the race had arrived there first and was waiting for me.

"Don't worry," he reassured me. "We'll cross together and I'll make sure you make it to the other side."

It took a little while for me to pluck up the courage to cross, but I knew I had to do it. I didn't want to drop out of the race, especially as I was on course to be the first female finisher. With Kenny's encouragement, I gripped his hand tightly and we plunged into the water together. We waded through with the water lapping at my thighs. It was rocky underfoot so I was concentrating as hard as I could on keeping my balance and squeezing his hand so much it must have hurt! I was petrified of falling over into the water and being swept away. It felt like it took an eternity to reach the other side of the bank but eventually we were there. I breathed a huge sigh of relief and could finally release the poor man from my vice-like grip.

He stayed with me for the remainder of the day, enabling me to have the courage to make it through all the other river crossings. His support and kindness is something I will never forget. I went on to be the first female finisher, and took fourth place overall. I was delighted I hadn't let the river crossings hold me back in the race, but they certainly didn't help alleviate my fear of water. If anything, they made it worse as I had memories of how fast the current had looked when the water swept around us. I was quite happy to keep on avoiding water as much as possible.

It was January 2018 when I finally plucked up the courage to have swimming lessons. At that point, I wasn't thinking about doing any swimming races or triathlons, I just wanted to face the fear that I had put off dealing with for so long. Learning to be able to do front crawl became my New Year's resolution. Once I set my mind to something, I become super-determined, so I told myself I would master this skill no matter what. This would push me way outside my comfort zone, so I kept in mind a quote by doctor, philosopher and author Debasish Mridha that has always resonated with me: "Comfort controls us. Fear scares us. To grow you have to overcome fear and go out of your comfort zone to be what you always wanted to be."

In order to make myself accountable to everyone so I couldn't back out of it, I put a post on Facebook telling all my followers I was going to learn how to swim. In response, a local triathlon coach, Kevin Draper, sent me a private message, kindly offering to give me lessons for free. I knew this was too good an opportunity to turn down. We arranged to have our first lesson at the leisure centre pool a week later. I nearly called him the evening before to cancel but I knew I would be letting down both him and myself if I didn't go. I told myself to be brave. I couldn't keep putting off dealing with my fears forever; the time had come to put on my big-girl pants!

That first lesson wasn't at all what I expected and I didn't do any actual swimming. Kevin could see how nervous I was when I arrived and assured me that we would take things slowly. He asked me to show him what I could do, and I instantly went into a panic and explained I could swim but only breaststroke with my head held firmly above the water. I told him I feared having my face submerged as it gives me a sensation of complete panic and a powerful surge of fear, making me almost hyperventilate. I explained that I would feel a shortness of breath as I couldn't get enough air into my lungs.

"Breathing is the key to being relaxed in the water," he told me as we stood in the shallow end. "So all I want you to do today is dip your head under the water and blow bubbles."

This sounded like a ridiculous idea, but I had total faith and trust in Kevin. Just dipping my face into the water sent a wave of panic over me. I immediately brought it back out again because I felt I couldn't breathe, even though it was only a matter of seconds that my face had been in the water. Gradually I began to feel slightly more relaxed and, with Kevin's guidance, we started practicing "sink downs". He told me it is important to learn how to do sink downs before you learn how to swim, as it teaches you to exhale in the water, making front crawl much easier and more relaxing.

At first it was a case of putting my head under water and blowing bubbles out, coming up, taking a breath, and going back down again. I didn't find it easy and I felt so silly. I can understand why Kevin uses this technique when he first teaches children to swim – they would find it great fun. We must have looked so funny to anyone watching – but I started not to care as much. In the past, I had become accustomed to people giving me funny looks when I was out running, dragging a tyre attached to my waist or with a heavy backpack to prepare for an ultra race. This was no different. With Kevin's encouragement, I was going underwater and slowly beginning to feel less panicked in the process. This was major progress for me. The more I did it, the less tense I became.

After the lesson I felt pure euphoria. It was that feeling of relief, pride and satisfaction that you get after achieving something you never thought you would be able to do. At that moment I was excited about my next lesson. But a week seemed to pass very quickly, by which time the excitement had disappeared, to be replaced once again with apprehension. Motivating myself to get into the car early in the morning and go to the pool was difficult, especially as it was cold and dark outside, but I knew Kevin would be waiting for me and I hate letting people down, especially if they are doing me a favour. It was too early to quit now.

The next lesson involved more sink downs but this time we moved to the middle of the pool, and then Kevin moved me up to the deep end. I kept close to the edge so if something happened, I knew I could grab onto the side and all would be well. Kevin demonstrated how it should be done as he sunk like a stone to the bottom of the pool.

"You made that look easy," I told him.

"Now it's your turn," he replied.

I took a breath in and let myself sink. As soon as my head was in the water I began to exhale, but I wasn't sinking like Kevin had: instead my body flipped over so my bottom came up to the surface. I was still exhaling at this point, then gradually began to sink but I only managed to get halfway to the bottom of the pool before coming up gasping for air.

"It is not as easy as you made it look!" I exclaimed to Kevin.

It took me several attempts before I could actually get my backside on the bottom of the pool. I obviously have a very buoyant body! It turns out that I wasn't exhaling enough, yet I was convinced I had blown every ounce of air out of my lungs.

Over the next few weeks, I worked incredibly hard as Kevin taught me how to do the front crawl. First he showed me how to use my arms correctly, then we practised my kicking. After that we put the arms, legs and breathing together. Coordinating it all was not easy. Over time, as I got the hang of the basics, we began to incorporate a few simple drills to help improve my technique. There was one particular drill I found extremely difficult called the 6-3-6 drill. This is where you are on your side, kick six times, take three strokes, breathe to one side, then kick another six times. I have extremely inflexible ankles, so my kick is very weak and, even though I think I am pointing my toes, I am not, which slows me down even more as I lose momentum. Swimming is all about technique and my natural instinct when taking a breath was to lift my head straight out of the water. This would make my feet sink and make swimming more difficult. Gradually I stopped lifting my head, learning how to rotate my body while swimming in order to be in the right position to breathe.

In between my lessons I had to go to the pool at least twice a week to practise. There were many occasions when I would get extremely frustrated with myself if I couldn't complete a task properly, or something I had found OK the week before I found tough the following week. Even the lifeguards started telling me not to be so hard on myself. They, and my fellow swimmers at the pool, were incredibly encouraging. I don't think they knew what a massive support they were to me at those times when I felt I couldn't do it or there seemed to be very little improvement.

In fact, Kevin told me my technique was getting better all the time, it was my lack of confidence and fear of not being able to breathe properly that were holding me back. He told me to start believing in myself more and not to compare myself to the other people I saw swimming effortlessly up and down the pool with grace and speed, making front crawl look simple. I had managed to believe in myself and not compare myself to others when it came to running but with swimming I found it much more difficult. Thankfully Kevin believed in me and his encouragement kept me going.

"You have come such a long way from being scared to even put your face in the water," he told me whenever I doubted my ability. "Don't be too hard on yourself or expect to see progress happening fast. I know you can succeed at whatever you set your mind to do and I have every confidence that you will be swimming lengths with ease in the future."

He was right. Thanks to his extraordinary patience and coaching, after a month of lessons I was able to complete nearly two lengths doing front crawl. It wasn't elegant; I started to lose my form towards the end, and I finished gasping for breath. But I didn't care. I had managed to complete almost two lengths. A month after that I achieved my biggest milestone – swimming four whole lengths (100 m) without stopping. I was so ecstatic afterwards, I wanted to dance around the changing room. I had felt the same way when I managed to complete a mile on the treadmill for the very first time. It was a very proud moment and something I never thought I would, or could, achieve. I had been sharing my progress on Instagram as I knew some of my followers had similar fears of water to me, so I couldn't wait to update my story to share the news. I simply couldn't stop grinning with excitement as I spoke to my followers from the changing room cubicle. Tim had been one of the people watching and when I got home, he had printed off a certificate saying I had completed my first 100 m swim. I proudly put it on the wall for everyone to see!

From then on my confidence grew and I was regularly swimming twice a week. I dreaded every session but afterwards I was always glad I had done it. Some weeks were good, others frustratingly difficult, but I kept plugging away. There was still lots of room for improvement when it came to my technique, but I was doing it and getting all the health and fitness benefits in the process. I was very proud of myself – yet I still felt my battle with my underwater demons wasn't won. Next, I had to conquer open-water swimming. Kevin suggested I come along on a Thursday evening to Weald Tri Club's regular open water swimming session, which took place at Bodiam Boating Station, Newenden, on the River Rother in Kent. I felt that old fear rising up inside me at just the thought of it and put off going several times. I simply couldn't face it, so I told Kevin I couldn't attend as I didn't have a wetsuit. Luckily – or unluckily depending on how you look at it – he very kindly said he could lend me an old one of his daughter's. Now I really had no excuse.

It still took me a few more weeks to pluck up the courage to turn up but, eventually, one sunny evening at the end of June 2018, I took the plunge. It didn't start well as I initially put my wetsuit on inside out. Thankfully, nobody else noticed but it did make me laugh! I walked to the end of the jetty and sat down, putting on my swim hat and goggles as I tried to psych myself up to slip into the murky water. My body seemed to have a mind of its own. I couldn't control the shaking and once again simply wanted to curl up in a ball and cry. Kevin was already in the water waiting for me and gave me plenty of reassurance as always. He told me we would ease into it just like I had in my very first pool lesson. All I had to do today was allow myself time to get used to being in the water and to adjust to the temperature, which was around 18°C (64°F). I didn't have to go straight into swimming, I just had to get my face wet and go back to the bubble blowing to regulate my breathing. Still I couldn't get in.

Kevin was incredibly patient as I hesitated, and told me my fears were perfectly normal when it came to open water swimming. Even confident and experienced pool swimmers could wobble on their first foray because it is such a different and unfamiliar environment compared to a clear, chlorine-filled pool. The water is colder and murkier, there are no lines on the bottom to follow, and swimming in a wetsuit can feel constrictive. Then there are the added fears of what might be in the water with you or lurking at the bottom. Kevin told me countless other swimmers had overcome these fears by gradual exposure to swimming in open water and that I would be the same.

I knew that if I didn't get in at that moment when it was totally safe then I would never conquer my fear. No one was expecting me to swim like a fish, all I had to do was get in and float. With a deep breath, I slid into the dark water. Everything inside me was telling me to get out and go home but Kevin simply told me to lie on my back and float – I could do that! Gradually I began to feel more comfortable floating. The next step was getting used to putting my face in the cold water and blowing bubbles. As soon as I tried, I instantly felt that sense of panic that I couldn't breathe. I was so surprised by the coldness of the water that I couldn't blow bubbles, so immediately took my face out of the water again. It took about 15 minutes until I felt a bit more relaxed and able to do it. Now it was time to see if I could swim! The moment my face went in and I began to do the front crawl was a real mixture of emotions. I couldn't see anything, I couldn't breathe, but I was doing it. After a few strokes I had to stop and regroup but I had taken the first step.

Over the following weeks, I kept going back and gradually gained in confidence. Kevin got me to keep swimming to different points along the river, getting further each time. I had lots of stops but the swimming sections were getting longer. Once again, I found it hard not to compare myself to others and I often felt demoralized when other swimmers would go zooming past me. Kevin reminded me to focus on what I was doing – not to compare – and to appreciate the progress I had made. From week to week I gained more confidence in the river, although there were often setbacks along the way when I doubted myself or felt too scared to carry on. Each time that happened, we would debrief, regroup and try again.

After several weeks of swimming in the river, I was then invited to join a few of the Weald Tri Club members who were going to Winchelsea to swim in the sea. This would be a huge test for me. I had slowly adjusted to swimming in the river, but would I be able to handle the currents and waves of the sea? The sea holds lots of bad memories in terms of swimming. Once when on holiday with Tim, he had been swimming in the sea while I was quite happily walking in the water with it only coming up as high as my chest. At that moment, I felt quite safe as I was able to stand and see the bottom. But then out of nowhere a large wave knocked me over, taking my feet from under me and lifting me out to sea. I felt as though I was being turned around and around like I was in a washing machine, I didn't know which way was up. Panic set in and I really didn't think I would be able to get back to the shore. After what seemed like ages, I was spat out of the current and able to touch the ground to walk free. I got out of the water as quickly as possible.

Luckily for me it was a hot and sunny day when we went to Winchelsea, otherwise I'm not sure I would have gone. From a distance, the water looked quite inviting and not too choppy. Tim and our Jack Russell terrier, Rani, came along for support and a walk, along with my friend Caroline, who is an avid swimmer. Once I had plucked up the courage to walk into the water, Rani came charging in after me. I'm not sure if this was because she was worried about me or didn't want to miss out on the fun and fancied a swim herself! It was very brave given she is so small and not usually a fan of water. After picking her up and going back to leave her safely with Tim, I realized as I headed back into the sea that I had to take a leaf out of Rani's book. I just had to charge into the water without thinking too much about it. Once again Kevin was there to guide me through the process. I seemed to swallow quite a lot of sea water, and I had a moment of panic when something unknown brushed past my leg. I didn't enjoy the way the waves were bouncing around me, particularly as they made it difficult to do the bilateral breathing technique Kevin had taught me. Every time I went to breathe on my right-hand side, I would be hit by a small wave so I found it easier to breathe on my left. It wasn't the most graceful of swims, but I did it. I swam in the sea. Another step forward.

CHAPTER NINE

TRI-ING SOMETHING NEW

Taking up cycling and swimming had opened up a whole new world for me, one I never expected to discover before I embarked on my run across America. By 2019, I was both swimming and cycling to a reasonable standard, I was able to run short distances again, and I had become a member of Weald Triathlon Club. So it made sense that I should actually try and complete a triathlon, even though the idea terrified me.

In April 2019, Kevin suggested I enter the Cranbrook Sprint Triathlon, which would take place at my local leisure centre that June. It would involve a 300-m (328-yd) swim, 21-km (13-mile) cycle and 5-km (3.1-mile) run. He said it was a good choice for my first attempt, as it was a small, friendly event close to home. There would be plenty of people from my tri club there to support me and it involved a pool swim, as opposed to a much more scary open-water one. I put off entering for ages but then decided I would go for it. I had no expectations on my finishing time; my aim was simply to finish, and to prove to myself in the process that I had overcome my fear of water.

As the swim would be started in waves of participants, I had to give a predicted swim time on my entry form. I was deliberately cautious about this. I didn't want to put myself under any extra pressure by being surrounded by faster swimmers. I wanted to be able to take my time, stay calm, and regulate my breathing. I wasn't going to be racing; I just wanted to complete the 300 m without having a panic attack.

I didn't do a great deal differently to prepare in terms of my training, although Kevin got me to practise swimming 200 m non-stop at the beginning of each of my lessons. I found this extremely tough so I couldn't imagine doing 300 m in one go in the race. I hoped I would find something extra on the day. The rest of the swim training remained the same, as did my cycling and twice weekly runs that included some speed training. I bought a triathlon suit to compete in and took it for a test swim at the pool to make sure it was comfortable. The benefit of having one of these is they can be worn for all three disciplines, saving time changing kit in transition. I needed all the help I could get to save time there. As you would expect of me, I originally wanted a pink tri suit, but then I realized that would make me stand out too much. I didn't want to draw extra attention to myself in case I ended up making any silly errors! I compromised by choosing a black one with a splash of pink and green at the end of each sleeve. I managed to add more pink by having a pink swimming cap and cycling helmet.

I'm a very organized person so the week before the event, I laid out all the kit I would need on the bed in the spare room ready to be packed into my bag, so I could keep double-checking it was all there and adding additional bits and pieces. As well as the tri suit, for the swim I needed a cap, goggles and towel. For the bike ride: cycling shoes, helmet, and, of course, the bike which I would pack on the day with a full water bottle on board and a bag with an emergency repair kit in case of punctures etc. As Mavis was set up on my turbo, I decided I would race on the latest addition to my bike collection, Pebbles. She's a gravel/adventure bike capable of performing on a variety of surfaces while still being comfortable. She can also be fitted with road tyres so I put those on for the triathlon as the bike route would all be on concrete. For the run, I needed trainers, sunglasses and a headband. I would also need some snacks that I would eat for energy between each discipline. I made the decision not to wear my knee support as it would take too much time to put it on between the cycle and the run. Although I had accepted my transitions wouldn't be fast, I still didn't want to be there all day. I also sometimes found if I didn't put the knee support on correctly first time it would rub on my shin bone so I would have to take it off and start again. I worried running without it could cause my knee to ache, but it was a chance I was going to have to take. I had also purchased a triathlon belt to attach my race number to – obviously I chose pink! This makes it easy to move the number so it is displayed on your back when cycling, and your front when running. My bike would have her own number attached to the frame. It was a lot to remember and I kept worrying I had forgotten something.

I only practised a transition once a few weeks before the race. I left my trainers on a bench in my garden, went for a 12-mile (19.3-km) ride and then returned home, dismounting my bike and running to the bench while removing my helmet. I tried to change my shoes as quickly as possible and then headed out on a 1-mile (1.6-km) run. Kevin had told me there were numerous ways I could shave a few seconds off my transition times, for example by having trainers with pull tight laces rather than the traditional lace ups. But as I wasn't bothered about going as fast as possible, I didn't feel extras like this were necessary for me. I knew my transitions weren't going to be slick, so I just wanted to keep things simple and familiar.

I got more and more anxious as race day approached and constantly wondered why I had signed up for it. Could I still pull out? One part of me really didn't want to do it. I was terrified about the swim, nervous about cycling in a competitive environment, and worried about running 3 miles without my knee support. But the other part of me knew how disappointed I would be with myself if I didn't go. If I stayed at home, I would be kicking myself for the rest of the day, and then somehow I would have to find the courage to enter another triathlon, most of which involved swimming in open water, which I definitely didn't feel ready for. Not only that, Kevin and my friends from the tri club were expecting to see me there. Others who followed me online were waiting to hear how I got on, as I had been sharing my triathlon journey on social media. A lovely lady called Pippa Cumbers had entered the Cranbrook Triathlon because of me so I definitely couldn't let her down by not turning up. I would have felt very embarrassed saying that I couldn't do it because I was too scared. I had to do this. I had worked too hard to quit now. After having one last wobble on the driveway before I left, I told Tim with determination: "I am going. I have to try."

"Good luck," he replied. "I'll see you there. I know you can do it."

He planned to catch up with me later to watch and cheer me on. I didn't share his confidence and for the entire drive there I was still battling my demons. I wanted to turn around and go home. But once I arrived, I saw a few friends getting their kit out of their cars who gave me a cheery wave and I started to feel a bit more at ease.

The next step was to register – where I discovered there was something I had forgotten: a hole punch! These are needed in order to attach your number to your tri belt. Who knew?! Thankfully someone else lent me theirs. With holes punched and my number attached, my next job was to rack up my bike in the transition area. Racking up the bike sounds like a simple job but it flummoxed me. Working out the best way to put the bike on the stand took some serious thought and I changed my mind several times about which would be the best way for her to face. As other people came and went leaving their bikes without hesitation, I realized I was over-thinking it. I pictured myself running from the pool and reaching for the bike. Was it better to have Pebbles with the front wheel facing me or facing away? In the end I opted for the front wheel to be facing me, racking it using the saddle. With the decision made, I laid out the rest of the kit I would need for the cycle and run on my towel close to the bike and then started chatting to some of the other competitors to stop me going back and changing my mind again.

My nerves increased as my start time drew closer. I was very concerned that the predicted time I had put for my swim was way too fast. Thankfully, I managed to make a last-minute change to my time slot. As we queued up to swim, we were given a timing chip that attached around our ankles. Watching the other participants in the water, it was a relief and a surprise to see lots of people doing breaststroke. I intended to try to front crawl the whole way as I had spent so long learning how to do it, but it was reassuring to know that breaststroke would be an option if I became too panicked about having my head in the water and being able to breathe. As I waited in line to start, my heart rate was through the roof. I attempted to do lots of relaxed breathing to calm myself down and tried to remember everything Kevin had taught me. I tried the best I could to avoid looking too much at the other competitors and comparing myself to them. They certainly looked more experienced than me. They looked like triathletes. But then I asked myself *what does a triathlete look like?* I knew full well that anyone of any body shape and size can be a triathlete. This was my time to become one. I knew I couldn't have been the only one there about to attempt a triathlon for the first time.

Once at the front of the line, you weren't allowed to dive in to start your swim. You had to get into the pool and wait at the end of the lane until the competitor in front had reached the shallow end. This was the most nerve-racking part for me. I was in the water and I knew I was shortly about to submerge my face and start swimming with more people around me than I had ever had before. It was terrifying. On top of my usual fears about swimming, I had the added pressure of being part of a race, and the associated expectations to perform well (although the only person putting such pressure on myself was me!). I had to keep telling myself to stay calm. I had to forget it was a race. It didn't matter about my time or my technique, I just had to be brave and get through it.

There was no more time to dwell on it as I heard the word "Go!" from the marshal who was setting me off. At that moment I saw Tim standing by the door where competitors exit the pool. Knowing he was there supporting me gave me the strength I needed. Now I couldn't fail! I took a deep breath and started swimming. My tactic was to not worry about speed and try to relax in the water. This hopefully would help to regulate my breathing. There were times when I felt other swimmers approaching from behind and I would start to feel panic rising up inside me but I knew I couldn't give in to it. I had to stay focused on what I was doing and not worry about anyone else.

Any fears of other competitors pulling at my legs and barging to get past were unfounded. Everyone was very polite and respectful. If you wanted to overtake a slower swimmer in the lane you were in, the rule was you tapped their foot and when you reached the end of the pool, the slower swimmer must let you pass. I allowed a couple of guys to go past me. They hadn't tapped my foot, but it made me feel less stressed to let them go ahead. I could feel my form going in the last couple of lengths, but I didn't care – I just needed to keep swimming, I was nearly there. Finally, I was on the last length. As I reached the end of the pool, the relief was enormous. The swim was over, I had done it! But I couldn't relax or celebrate yet. There was still the bike ride and run to do.

I climbed up the steps, missing the lower rung of the ladder the first time I tried as I was rushing to get out. I walked with speed to the door, then once outside I ran towards the transition area while taking off my goggles and swimming cap. But where was my bike?! In the sea of other bikes all racked up and waiting to be ridden, I couldn't see Pebbles at all. I had even practised running from the door to my bike before the triathlon started, but I still couldn't remember where I had left her. Thankfully Tim and my friend Evie who had joined him had spotted her.

"Mimi she's over here!" they yelled at me, pointing.

I dashed underneath a line of bikes and then I finally spotted Pebbles waiting for me. Everything that happened next felt as though it was happening in slow motion. Other participants were coming and going at speed while the transition seemed to be taking me ages. I sat down to put my cycling shoes on, and as I did so I knocked the next-door bike, nearly causing a domino effect. Thankfully a fast-reacting competitor grabbed the bike before it fell over and crashed into the other bikes, sparing me from any further blushes. I dried my feet and put on socks (which I found out later I shouldn't have bothered doing), put on my cycling shoes and helmet, then grabbed Pebbles, pushing her at a jog towards the start of the cycle leg. At that moment, I actually felt I looked like I knew what I was doing!

Once I reached the blue line, T1 (transition one) was over and I was able to get onto Pebbles for the start of the cycle section. All my fears from the swim had disappeared; I was in my element and loved this stage. It was a good, solid 21 km (13 miles) of cycling. Every time I saw someone ahead, I did my best to overtake; I guess I can't always switch off my competitive nature! Before I knew it, I had completed the distance and it was back into transition two, where I left Pebbles behind, changed into my trainers and headed out for the start of the run.

I had been warned that lots of people find it tough finding their running legs after being on the bike. In the first minute of the run, I struggled to catch my breath, perhaps because I was trying to rush to make up some time that I had lost in transition. My legs felt good, but my lungs simply didn't seem to be working, leaving me with no option but to walk for a minute to try and regulate my breathing. Once I was ready to go again, I felt much better. Up ahead I saw that my friend Bonita, who I had overtaken at the end of the bike ride, had pulled away from me again, so I ran to catch her up and overtake.

It wasn't an easy course as most of the run was off road and hilly, but I just kept putting one foot in front of the other. The route was out and back, and I loved saying "hi" to all the other runners coming towards me. The fastest competitors zoomed by looking fantastic, pushing themselves to the finish line and glory. As I could only do a couple of runs per week, in contrast to them my pace wasn't that fast, but I wasn't bothered. I was enjoying the moment and hoping my knee would hold up. I wasn't in it to win it, I was here to enjoy taking part and I was certainly doing that. I loved being on my home turf as I kept seeing people I knew who were either supporting, marshalling or taking part. After all my worries a few hours earlier, it felt great to be part of an event again. It was a fantastic feeling to be back running. I didn't feel any discomfort in my knee till near the end. Knowing how much pain I had been able to run through in America, I knew I would be able to finish now.

Heading towards the finish line on the home straight felt fantastic. I was grinning from ear to ear as I knew I had done it. I gave a big wave to Tim as I spotted him on the side of the road proudly filming me. As I passed him, he then had to make a mad dash to capture me crossing the finish line. As I reached the line I threw my arms up in the air in triumph. I had done it! I was ecstatic. I was now a triathlete! This is a title I never thought I would hold. I never believed I would have the courage or ability to do it because of the swim. Being a member of Weald Tri Club had made such a huge difference to me. Being surrounded by friends gave me confidence and I was grateful for their support. After chatting with friends at the finish line to compare race notes, I was reunited with Tim who gave me a big hug. I proudly showed him the medal. This was one to treasure. It might not have been as long as some of my other events, or as painful, but I felt this was right up there with my other achievements.

Results were soon available, and my times weren't anything special but that didn't bother me. I could see where there was plenty of room for improvement – especially in the transitions. I went home to have a bath followed by a glass or two of bubbles to celebrate. A few hours later a friend sent me a message to say I had actually won my age category. I couldn't believe it! I hadn't stayed for the presentation as I never expected to win anything. More good news came when I found out my friend Pippa had come third in her age category. Once my trophy and a chocolate prize had been passed on to me, I shared a picture of it on my social media accounts to thank those who supported me. I was touched afterwards to hear from Susie, part of the film crew who travelled with me across America, who messaged to congratulate me.

She told me: "Well done on your first triathlon! I know you're not a confident swimmer and now you're kicking even more ass!" Catching me up on her news, she added: "I have felt very empowered since the trip across America and from watching you deal with everything that you did. Now when I face any challenges my mantra has become: 'Mimi ran fifty-seven miles in a day, I think you can manage this!' You're an inspiration." Susie's words meant a lot to me. I hoped my experience would show others what is achievable if you put your mind to it and put the training in. There were so many times I had wanted to give up as I found it all so overwhelming, but now I was a triathlete, and I had a trophy to prove it!

CHAPTER TEN

MY NEW SPORTING FUTURE

When the surgeons suggested after America that I would be able to find sporting fulfilment away from ultrarunning, I didn't believe them. But after completing the Ride Across Britain I finally found a love for cycling. I had got the cycling bug and I was keen to do more events. After doing some research into various challenges, I decided sticking to long distance rides was the way I wanted to go, rather than doing lots of Sportives (races). The latter tend to be more competitive with detailed published results, prizes for the fastest riders and time pressure to complete each stage.

I had intended to have more adventures with my running rather than racing after America, so it seemed natural that I would want to do events that were challenging but not competitive in cycling too. In 2019, I took part in a number of organized rides in the UK, ranging in distance from 66 to 192 miles (106 to 309 km). I also loved doing a couple of self-organized long-distance rides with friends, including cycling around the Isle of Wight with Caroline and riding 328 miles (528 km) from Land's End to Bristol with Becky.

In August 2019, I took part in the popular Prudential Ride London, a 100-mile (161-km) loop from London to Surrey as it's part of the "London Classics" challenge. You have to complete the bike ride, run the London Marathon, and swim 2 miles in the Serpentine in Hyde Park in order to win a special medal. The events can be completed in any order over any time period. I ran the London Marathon back in 2005 so completing the bike ride would take me two thirds of the way there.

I'm glad I had the experience of taking part in Ride London, as it is one of the most famous mass participation bike events in the UK, but I have to admit it wasn't my favourite cycling experience. I enjoyed chatting to lots of new people, especially when we were held at the start in pens to go off in waves, but the large numbers made the course congested. There were times when there were so many people, bottlenecks would appear, and we had to get off our bikes. On two occasions I had to walk for half an hour or more. I found this stop-starting quite frustrating. Luckily, I managed to get to, and over, Box Hill without any problems as well as Leith Hill. Others weren't so lucky as they missed the cut-off due to time constraints, or because there were too many people going up at the time, so they had to be diverted along a slightly shortened route. I would have been miffed if that had happened to me, especially if

I had missed the cut-off because of something that was out of my control.

In all the cycling events I have done, I've enjoyed the fact there was no pressure. I wasn't taking part to try to win or get a placing. Cycling for me is more about completing than competing, whereas with running, I was more competitive. When cycling, I prefer to enjoy the experience and adventure of a long bike ride without any pressure to finish in a certain time or position. Even if I had wanted to be competitive, I don't feel I have the talent or potential to be one of the best. I just want to enjoy being out on my bike. There is plenty I can do to improve but my desire to be better isn't because I want to gain fast times or podium placings. It is so I can become more experienced and confident, allowing me to see more places and have more adventures. I also feel being a competitive cyclist is much harder than being a competitive runner as there are so many other variables involved. There is so much that can go wrong in a cycling race compared to running – your chain could snap, you could get a puncture, there could be a crash between competitors. I feel more in control when running, as it is just me, not me and my bike.

* * *

While I enjoyed taking part in all these bike rides, what I was really craving was a bigger adventure. I had loved travelling the world when I was running, exploring new places and covering long distances in the process. I thrived on having something challenging to prepare for, not just physically but planning a route and all the little things to consider along the way to make it a success. So I decided to go back to America in September 2019 and cycle the Pacific Coast Highway. The route takes in what is said to be one of the most spectacular coastlines in the world so I knew I would be guaranteed a ride with amazing views.

With running I didn't mind having these experiences on my own but, with cycling, I prefer to have company and to be able to share the journey with someone else. I was delighted when my friend Catriona Archer agreed to take time off work to join me. She is a much more experienced cyclist than me which would be helpful. I just hoped I would be able to keep up with her, especially on the hills, as she's a total powerhouse on the climbs!

The route would involve cycling 1,867.5 miles (3,004.4 km) with a cumulative elevation of 91,677 ft (27,943 m) over 25 days. Some of this would be on traffic-free cycle paths and other sections along main roads. We would start in Vancouver, Canada, then travel down the West Coast of America till we reached the Mexican border. I would have to pack light as we would have to carry everything we needed on our bikes. This included our tents as we would be camping at sites we could find along the route. I felt that buzz of excitement I used to get ahead of my ultra challenges as I pored over maps to plot our daily distances and find places where we could stay each night. Cat also suggested that a website she had used before called Warm Showers could come in useful. It is a community of cyclists who offer rooms in their homes for people to stay in when on cycling expeditions. My personal preference was to camp, but it was good to have this as an option if we were stuck for somewhere to stay.

I had to research the best kit to ensure my bags were light, while still making sure I had all the essentials. As with any plan, I knew it would have to be flexible as there could be unexpected hiccups along the way. But, whatever happened, we needed to complete the journey in exactly 25 days due to the limited time Cat could take off work. To do this, we would have to cycle an average of 74 miles per day.

I would be riding the Highway on Pebbles as she can be fitted with wider tyres to make the journey more comfortable and her gearing is fantastic. She is much lighter than my hybrid and can be fitted with a rack on the back of the bike to carry panniers. All in all, she would be ideal for this trip. In the build-up, I did several days of consecutive long rides to replicate what I would be doing on the Pacific Coast Highway. I practised riding with the panniers on my bike, making the bags heavier as the weeks went by, so I could get used to cycling with the extra weight. It wasn't easy to begin with and I felt extremely unbalanced, but I soon got used to it.

My confidence took a bit of a knock a month before I was due to fly to Canada when I came off Pebbles in spectacular style. I was cycling on a loop near my house when I went around a tight bend on a narrow road at the same time as a van was coming the other way. I didn't have much time to react and swerve out of the way which caused me to lose control, fly off my bike, and land at the side of the road with my bike on top of me. Thankfully I didn't seem to be badly hurt, and Pebbles wasn't damaged, but I came away feeling quite shocked, battered and bruised with very sore ribs. Cycling home was extremely painful as I couldn't get my breath. I discovered later that I had fractured a rib. Mentally it made me more fearful about cornering on such narrow lanes, but it didn't put me off wanting to cycle. After a couple of days' rest I was back on Pebbles – but I decided to stay away from the loop where I crashed just in case! I think what shocked and upset me the most about the accident was that the van driver didn't stop to check if I was OK. They must have known it had happened but continued down the lane without a second thought.

I was relieved to have physically recovered by the time we were due to start cycling the Pacific Coast Highway and I put any fears of crashes or falls to one side, focusing instead on the exciting adventure that lay ahead of us. It started the day before the ride when we met up with an old school friend of mine, Chris Rogers, and her husband, who took Cat and I on a sightseeing tour of Vancouver. The highlight was visiting Stanley Park in the downtown area of the city. It is a natural West Coast rainforest with the Vancouver

Harbour on one side and Strait of Georgia on the other. It was amazing going from the busy, built-up urban area full of skyscrapers straight into this tranquil, green oasis. The huge cedar, maple and fir trees were magnificent to see while the views across the still waters were breathtaking.

It's the perfect place for a run, I thought. If my body was able, I could run around this spectacular park all day. But I had our adventure on two wheels to look forward to instead.

We set off from Vancouver at 6 a.m. on 3 September. It felt fantastic to be embarking on this incredible journey. We were feeling fresh and full of energy – but we soon encountered some extremely steep hills, which were made even more difficult to climb by our heavy bikes laden down with luggage. It was easier (but still hard work!) to dismount and push our bikes up the steepest parts. Just before lunch we crossed the border into America which felt very exciting; I had never crossed a controlled border on foot/cycle before. It was also a bit confusing. When we arrived, there were loads of queues of cars as well as a few pedestrians. We weren't sure which line we should join as cyclists. A helpful border guard soon ushered us into a building where we could show our passports. It was all very efficient, so we were quickly on our way again. It was hard to tell we were in a new country to begin with as, unsurprisingly, the scenery looked just like it had in Canada.

After a quick bite to eat at a gas station we passed, we carried on to Bay View in the state of Washington to camp for the night. Unfortunately, during the 90 miles (145 km) we had pedalled that day, we hadn't found anywhere to buy food for our supper so we ended up feasting on a packet of tortilla chips. Not ideal given all the calories we were burning in the saddle. If only I could have brought Jan along with me on this trip to cook for us!

We were starving when we set off the next morning, but thankfully we soon passed a cafe where we stopped for breakfast. We planned to cycle 45 miles (72 km) to Port Townsend. Some of this route was on cycle paths but on other sections we had to travel along busy roads. There was a big hard shoulder but there were still some pretty scary moments when drivers would get too close when overtaking. This brought back memories of my run across America and how nervous I would feel about vehicles whizzing by in such close proximity to me. On the plus side, the roads were a lot smoother than those I was used to cycling on in England, so at least I didn't have to worry about potholes all the time.

We had to catch a ferry across a bay to reach Port Townsend where we set up camp for the night in Fort Worden Historical State Park. The fort on the site was an active US Army base between 1902 and 1953 so was once buzzing with soldiers. It was first constructed in 1898 as part of a coastal defence system known as "The Triangle of Fire". Today it's a state park where you can enjoy picturesque hiking trails, tour the historical military buildings and enjoy the views of the surrounding sea.

There is a huge campsite in the park, so it was a no-brainer to make this beautiful and interesting location one of our overnight stops. I had decided in advance to bring a free-standing tent which was a great call as it was much easier to put up than one needing to be held up by guy ropes and tent pegs, particularly as the ground was very hard here. As it was only our second night, I was still getting used to erecting my tent in the quickest way possible but I hoped by the end of the trip I would be doing it in seconds.

We knew conditions the next day would be more challenging when we continued south, hugging the coastline, because we kept passing signs warning of "severe side winds ahead". I worried about being blown into the path of traffic. We must have timed it well, though, to avoid the winds at their worst as it didn't seem too bad, and I was always in control of Pebbles. The winds did pick up overnight, which made it difficult to sleep as my tent sides rattled noisily with every gust. Still awake in the early hours, I had to get up and go for a pee. I was annoyed about having to get up until I saw the stunning night sky outside my tent. I was greeted by thousands of twinkling stars shining against a jet-black sky that stretched above me. I could see many different constellations and I suddenly felt a pang of emotion that Tim wasn't with me. He would have been able to tell me exactly what they all were. As usual, he had been incredibly supportive of my desire to come on this trip, even though it meant being away from home for a month.

The next morning we awoke to find two other female cyclists had arrived during the night and we soon got chatting to them. They were called Ryan and Darin and we were amazed to hear they were coming to the end of a bike ride that had taken them around the world. They were finishing their journey along the Highway to return to their homes in California. As we were heading in the same direction, we spent some of the day cycling with them and they were wonderful company.

The next day the opening miles we had to cover weren't very undulating, so we made good progress. I knew despite all my planning that we should expect the unexpected – and that happened when we reached the place where I had intended for us to camp for the night. We got there only to find no campsite existed. We decided to carry on and later stumbled upon an RV park with available tent pitches which had a pool and a jacuzzi, making the extra unplanned miles that day well worth it.

By day six we reached the state of Oregon. I had been told this was an area of amazing natural beauty and it didn't disappoint. It was mile after mile of stunning scenery including craggy coastal pines and amazing rock formations in the sea. As we weren't racing or up against the clock, we could take our time and we often stopped to enjoy the views and take a few pictures. I loved looking out across the water, seeing boats bobbing in harbours and quaint, traditional lighthouses. The sea was often incredibly flat, so it was very peaceful to just sit and watch it for a short time before getting back in the saddle.

The weather had been pretty kind to us so far but when we travelled towards the city of Astoria, it started tipping it down. At this point we were cycling along a very busy road which was my worst nightmare. Lorries were thundering past at high speed, and I could barely see where I was going as the raindrops were stabbing me in the eye. Cat was cycling behind me and told me later that some of the lorries looked like they were very close to me even though I was on the hard shoulder.

Another terrifying element of this section was having to cycle through a number of long tunnels. There was a button we had to press at the entrance to each tunnel that lit up warning signs throughout to alert drivers to our presence. There wasn't a huge amount of room to move out of the way if they hadn't seen us. Even though I hoped drivers would be proceeding more carefully because they had been warned we were there, I still felt like I was holding my breath the entire way through and let out a huge sigh of relief when we made it out the other side. Thankfully we were soon back to quieter roads and cycle paths with amazing sea views. There were plenty of steep hills and I found I was getting more confident on the descents as the journey went on. I still couldn't keep up with Cat though, who would whizz down them without any fear.

As we approached a place called Depoe Bay, we were surprised to see a crowd of people staring out at the sea. We couldn't resist stopping to see what they were looking at and I'm so glad we did. They were whale watching. It was a treat to see the grey whales breaking out above the surface of the water and then dipping back down with their tails arching behind them. Further along the Oregon coast, we were able to catch a glimpse of a few sea lions sunning themselves on a large rock.

While the scenery and wildlife we had encountered so far were spectacular, we were struggling when it came to finding decent food. We often had to resort to disgusting sandwiches from the small supermarkets and petrol stations we passed. Coming across a larger supermarket or an independent store selling fresh produce was always a cause for celebration. It was just a shame we could never carry much on our bikes to take forwards on the journey with us.

By day ten my body was holding up really well. The only slight soreness I was getting was towards the end of each day, when the ball of my foot started hurting from being clipped into the pedals for so long. It was an uncomfortable but manageable pain, so I didn't let it bother me. It always went away as soon as I stopped and unclipped. I was relieved I wasn't having any more major aches and pains. Sadly, the same couldn't be said for Pebbles. I started having issues with the gears which were getting increasingly difficult to change. We passed a bike shop in the city of Bandon,

Oregon, where we decided to stop and get her checked out. It's just as well we did as they told us there wouldn't be another bike shop on our route for at least 100 miles (161 km). It turned out my chain and cassette all needed to be changed as they had worn out. Luckily I had caught it in time before it completely broke when we were on the road.

As we continued on our final section of the Oregon coastline towards the city of Brookings, the coastal views just got better and better. I have never seen so many amazing shades of blue. The sea sparkled in different colours as the sun shone on it and changed shade as the waves lapped up to the shore. As it stretched off to the horizon it met the huge sky in another beautiful blue which was dotted with fluffy, white clouds.

On day 12 we rode out of Oregon and into California. Just like on my run across the US, crossing a state line always gave me a thrill and felt like a real achievement. We didn't see much of California to begin with as it was a very misty morning with the clouds shrouding our view. Thankfully it had cleared by the time we reached our first forest of Redwood trees. I had been excited about seeing these green giants since planning the trip, and they were just as breathtaking as I had expected. They are the tallest living things on our planet, growing 300 to 350 feet (90 to 107 m) tall and 16 to 18 feet (4.9 to 5.5 m) across. I felt very small in comparison to these beautiful, majestic trees and it was a privilege to cycle beneath them.

At our campsite the next morning, I was woken by a funny, snuffling noise going on outside my tent. On investigation, I discovered a raccoon eating some peanut butter which he had stolen from one of Cat's bike bags. The clever rascal knew how to take the lid off with its paws and was tucking in like Winnie the Pooh with a pot of honey. It was hilarious – but we were also furious as we needed that peanut butter for breakfast. I shooed him off only for a skunk to then come and try his luck a few moments later. When we were packed up and on our way again, we were treated to more Redwoods as we passed through what is known as the "Avenue of Giants" in Humboldt Redwoods State Park. Once again, it was marvellous and humbling to pedal past the massive trunks and high green branches that stretched up into the sky. I felt like a tiny ant beneath them.

I woke up on day 14 feeling slightly nervous; we were headed to a place called Leggett at 984 feet (300 m) above sea level, which was going to include our longest climb. Once the incline began, although it was tough, it was nowhere near as bad as I thought it would be. The worst bit was coming down the other side as there were some tight hairpin turns where I feared I might crash if I couldn't make the turning in time and stay in control. I was fine though – and I even managed to overtake a couple of other cyclists we passed which I felt rather smug about. It seems my competitive spirit is never far away!

For the next few days the route continued to be very undulating as we were in the mountainous region of Mendocino County. The ups and downs were relentless. I found it especially tough as my gears were playing up again and the chain kept slipping when I tried to change them. I vowed to get them looked at again at the earliest opportunity. One section was particularly frightening as there was a massive drop on one side of the narrow road and the conditions were foggy. When it cleared and I had the confidence to look up from the road ahead, there were some glorious views of the coast below.

The next highlight of the trip was reaching San Francisco and cycling over the Golden Gate Bridge. I had driven across it once before on a holiday with Tim and would never have imagined that one day I would be back, travelling across the iconic mile-long suspension bridge on a bike. We had found a bike shop shortly beforehand where a particularly grumpy man had been able to fix my gears. I had been starting to feel a little fatigued as we had ticked off some 80-mile (129-km) days over hilly terrain, so passing through San Francisco invigorated me. I was loving this adventure so much. As we carried on further south into California, we now had many more options along the way for places to stop to eat and drink. I felt as though I was eating like a horse, enjoying BLTs and fries, plus copious amounts of delicious ice cream, but I had still lost a bit of weight. This didn't concern me though; it had often happened to me during running challenges and I always put it on again afterwards.

We had used the Warm Showers website to stay with hosts on a couple of nights so far. Everyone we met was very warm and accommodating. They often treated us to some wine and let us use their washing machines to clean our kit. It was nice to be able to sleep in a bed rather than the hard ground, but I did prefer camping in general as I felt a little intrusive being in the homes of people we had never met before.

By week three, we were passing through Santa Barbara, which is nicknamed the "American Riviera" because of its vineyards and Mediterranean-style architecture. I was delighted when we reached a bridge with a button for us to push before crossing which lit up a sign telling drivers there was a "Bicyclist on Bridge". I have always called myself a "bicyclist" so I felt as though the sign was there especially for me!

The next section of our route took us slightly inland to find the campsite where we planned to stay for the night. On our way there, we passed numerous fruit farms and even a few cannabis fields. Cat was cycling ahead of me and for some reason her GPS took her in completely the wrong direction. I shouted and shouted for her to stop and turn back to no avail as she couldn't hear me. I stopped and sent her a text message hoping she wouldn't go too far off course before she saw it. It wasn't long till she realized I wasn't behind her and she checked her phone to see my message. Reunited, we made it to the campsite for a much-needed sleep.

It was then on to Malibu and L.A. heading towards San Diego. This section of coast had some beautiful sandy beaches lined with palm trees and harbours full of huge superyachts. The route was mostly cycle paths which I much preferred to being beside traffic. At one point the cycle path actually passed right through the middle of a sandy beach – which was bizarre but wonderful. The temperature started heating up, so we often rode in just a vest and shorts. I loved feeling the Californian sun on my back. We finished the day just outside Laguna Beach having covered 95 miles (153 km).

The next day was our last. In between cycling, we had to catch another ferry across San Diego Bay which was packed full of fellow cyclists. Then it was on to the Mexican–United States border, which we couldn't miss as President Trump's controversial wall had been built there. Reaching the wall between the two countries, we dismounted our bikes and hugged in celebration. Both of us felt a massive sense of achievement having reached the Mexican border after starting our journey in Canada. Despite the odd puncture, my gear woes and once or twice accidentally going off-course, we had stuck to our plan and finished the route in 25 days. I loved every moment; it was an extraordinary experience and, just like my run across America, a unique way to see such a beautiful part of the world. Once again, it opened my eyes to how vast and varied the continent is.

Despite all the miles we had covered, I felt as though I could have carried on if needed which was a good sign. Our longest day in the saddle was about 97 miles (156 km) and our shortest was around 48 miles (77 km). Cat and I had got on well despite spending 24/7 together and agreed we would do more long-distance rides in the future. I returned home feeling uplifted by the whole experience and ready to take on more adventures on my bike. Sadly, the ones I had planned for 2020 had to be postponed due to the Coronavirus pandemic. I felt very lucky during lockdown that we were still able to go outside to exercise – even though this was limited to once a day initially. Going out on my bike then became even more valuable to my mental and physical health. I was also grateful to have my turbo so I could cycle at home. When races and travel can resume, I'm looking forward to doing more adventures; I'm currently planning one with a friend, which I'm beyond excited about. It will involve the pair of us cycling self-supported across a continent.

Although at first it didn't fill my heart with as much joy as running, I have grown to love cycling. I will now spend hours cycling outside or inside on the turbo. I definitely feel as though I'm a bona fide cyclist now, as I have a bike for all occasions! As well as Marv, Mavis and Pebbles, I have a fourth bike, Sylvia, an Avail Advanced Pro 1. I was lucky enough to be asked to try her out by the brand Liv Cycling UK. It is designed specifically for women and this particular model is an endurance road bike. Perhaps I would have learned to love cycling earlier in my life if I had found a bike that is as perfect a match for me as Sylvia.

Now I am cycling so much, I have been asked by many people if I would go back and redo my run across America on the bike. Would it put some ghosts to rest to complete the route by cycling? The answer is no. For starters, the route I ran would not be suitable to cycle on, as some of it involved very technical terrain. And many of the road sections would be too dangerous to cycle on too. I also have no desire to return to New York. It is not a place filled with happy memories for me. There are many other new places I would rather explore and discover instead. Carol has suggested creating a virtual version of the route that people could run or cycle when the documentary is released (currently this is planned for 2021). I would be more tempted to cycle it this way.

If I were to return to America with my bike for a big challenge, the one that interests me is cycling the TransAmerica Bicycle Trail. It is another West- to East-coast route that starts in Oregon and finishes 4,228 miles (6,804 km) later in Virginia, passing through ten states along the way. I watched a documentary about it and thought it looked like an amazing experience. The top riders finish in about 16 days, while others can take up to 70, or as long as you want. It is a self-sufficiency event where cyclists have to carry all their kit, keeping everything as minimal as possible. It is this kind of ride that really appeals to me rather than racing, and it would be another wonderful way to see America. I just need to convince someone to do it with me!

Just like when I first took up running, I am enjoying learning about what cycling has to offer, seeing new places, and pushing myself to see what I am capable of. I might not be able to run long distances any more, but I feel very lucky that I can still have adventures on two wheels rather than two feet.

* * *

I have also grown to enjoy swimming more than I ever expected. More than two years on from the start of my journey, where all I could do was blow bubbles into the water, I can't believe how far I have come. I can now do front crawl. I have swum in rivers and the sea. And I swam in a competitive environment to become a triathlete. I still don't feel like a natural swimmer, though, and I get frustrated with myself because I find it difficult to breathe if I don't stay relaxed. Even now, I have slight anxiety with my breathing which means somewhere deep down inside me I'm still holding on to the fear of water. But it is receding as time goes on. I knew it was going to take time to overcome my fear as it is so deep-seated from my childhood.

I never thought I would be able to put on a wetsuit and go swimming in open water so I am very proud I can do that now. Although I often still feel fearful about putting my face in the water as a wave of panic hits me, I have started to enjoy elements of wild swimming, such as being immersed in nature on a tranquil summer's day and swimming with friends. There are times when I have had swans glide past me, flocks of geese fly over me and swallows swoop by. Or I have swum past some beautiful flowers blooming on the riverbank. Occasionally the odd fish will leap out of the water.

During the Coronavirus lockdown, open-water swimming was permitted before indoor swimming pools reopened, so the fact I had learned to do it meant I had another exercise option during this time of confinement. I was secretly quite pleased when the leisure centre pools remained closed for so long. Even though I had been enjoying pool swimming more than I used to, it was still not something I looked forward to. I was also quite relieved when the September 2020 Swim Serpentine event was cancelled after I had entered. I wasn't sure I was quite ready for a 2-mile (3.2-km) open-water swim. I will pluck up the courage to do it another year though, so I can complete the London Classics challenge.

The summer of 2020 was a good one for me in terms of swimming, because there was no pressure to race, so all my trips to the river were with the sole goal of learning how to relax in the water. This then helps with my breathing.

Although I still haven't mastered it, I am getting better. Recently I met a couple of guys who regularly swim 2 miles in the river and one of them always wears a nose clip. He told me that without one, his nose would stream for hours after swimming. This also happened to me so I ordered a pink one to see if it would make a difference. It definitely has stopped my nose from running afterwards and has also unexpectedly helped with my breathing. Now I can concentrate on blowing air out of my mouth when underwater, rather than out of my nose and mouth.

I might not be passionate about swimming, but I am proud and pleased that I can do it now. I have been able to conquer my lifelong fear of water in my fifties, which shows it is never too late to put the past to bed, or to learn new skills.

* * *

When it comes to running, I'm pleased I can now run two, sometimes three times a week. The longest I usually do is 6 miles (9.7 km) and the others are 3 to 5 miles (4.8 to 8 km). Any more than that and I can feel my knee starting to hurt so I don't try to push it. I very much listen to my body, so I am happy not to run for a week to give my knee a rest if needed. I know there is the possibility of running another half marathon in the future but, at this stage, I wonder whether it is worth it because of the impact it will have on my knee. The training involved and the race itself would likely set my knee back again and lead to me needing to have an extended period of rest. At the moment, I would prefer to keep running consistently, rather than trying to do more and then needing extra downtime to recover. I know other people who have tried to run through similar knee problems to mine, and they end up not enjoying the races they have entered and having very stop-start training. I'm not bothered about doing many competitive races in the future as I know I won't be able to go as fast as I used to. I love taking part in my local parkrun, and volunteering for them. I might never beat my quickest time there of 22.01 but I can still try and improve my current time, and just enjoy running with others.

I'm lucky that I was able to take part in many of the world's best ultra races – such as Badwater, Comrades and Spartathlon – during my ultrarunning days. I ran most of the races on my bucket list so I have no regrets. I'm sure if I could still run long distances, I would have found more races I wanted to do, as new ones pop up all the time. But my plan after America had always been to have more adventures running in different places around the world, rather than trying to gain more PBs or world records; after all, running should be fun.

In 2019, my JOGLE world record was broken after 11 years. I am surprised and delighted to have held it for that long. If I were still able to run that far in such a short period of time (840 miles / 1,352 km in just over 12 days), I certainly wouldn't have gone back to try again. I feel I have been there, done that and got the record. I never expected to have it forever. I strongly believe records are there to be broken and I was only looking after it until someone better came along. In 2020 it was broken again.

The more time I have spent away from ultrarunning, the less I have missed it. I have found there are other ways I can still stay involved. I continue to give my inspirational talks, sharing my experiences at festivals, in schools and at corporate events. The feedback I get is incredibly rewarding as people tell me I have inspired them to take up running or do their first ultra. I am also giving something back by crewing for friends. In July 2018, Tim and I crewed for my friend Debbie King at the Badwater Ultra. I was her head crew which was a massive responsibility. My job was to ensure she got to the finish line in the portals of Mount Whitney within the cut-off time and ensure her and the rest of her crew's safety while we were in one of the hottest places in the world.

I didn't mind that I wasn't racing it myself as I had taken part twice before. It was wonderful to be there to support my friend and see her achieve something she had spent seven years working towards. I did the most running I had done for a while supporting Debbie and I loved it. Watching her cross the finish line was extremely emotional, and it felt very special to have been part of it. Then in August 2018, I was able to turn the tables with Becky and crew for her while she ran the North Downs Way 100, her first 100-

mile (161-km) race. I loved helping her achieve her goal and seeing her finish after everything she has done for me.

There have also been ultra races around the world I have had the privilege to help stage. In April 2018, I was asked to go to Fiji to be the Race Director for a new ultra, set up by Wes Crutcher, called the Lost Island Ultra. How often do you get the chance to go to a tropical island in the South Pacific? I jumped at the chance and felt extremely excited and privileged to be part of this inaugural event. It is a 137-mile (220-km) race in five-day stages on marked trails with amazing views. My role was to support Wes, so I would look after the runners ensuring that they were happy, and give a few of the race briefings in the mornings. I would be present along the course to deal with any issues and then be at the finish at the end of each day to greet all the runners as they came in. I felt I was up to the task thanks to my running experience of multi-day events. I would have a few nuggets of wisdom to give, while also having a lot to learn! It was a wonderful experience but challenging at times thanks to the conditions. The course had to be changed at the last minute as a destructive cyclone had passed through a couple of days before the start, causing some of the intended paths to become inaccessible. Another cyclone was forecast the day we were scheduled to finish, so we couldn't take any chances of it over-running. On the final stage, runners ran through the majestic Sigatoka Sand Dunes National Park for a final sprint along the beach to cross a unique finish line – which was in the sea! It was an honour to see the fantastic group of runners finish. I felt very emotional for them. Luckily everyone did finish just before the second cyclone hit the island.

In stark contrast to the tropics I went to the Arctic Circle the following year, as Tim and I crewed for runners in the 6633 Arctic Ultra. I had run (and won) this 352-mile (566-km) self-sufficiency race in 2007 so I knew exactly what the competitors would be going through (although the route is now slightly different from the one I did). You have to pull everything you need in your own sled and the biggest challenge is avoiding hypothermia in the freezing conditions. It was wonderful to return to this part of the world where the frozen landscape is simply spectacular. Emily Like (the race director's daughter) and I would go out each day when the athletes were on the course and do our own walk of 6 miles or more, depending on how much time we had. It was very special being on the ice road once again. It was when I was racing here in 2007 that my father sadly passed away so returning was extremely emotional. When I reached the point on the ice road where I had been when I had felt he had died, I stood quietly with tears streaming down my face while I had a lovely chat with him in my head. Helping all the runners complete their epic journey in the Arctic was wonderful, emotional and inspiring.

Another way I am keeping in touch with the ultrarunning world is via online coaching. I love helping my athletes achieve their goals. It is extremely rewarding, and I can live vicariously through their experiences and achievements.

While there are of course times I still miss ultrarunning, I am very grateful for the fact I can put my trainers on and go for a run, whether that is for 6 miles, 3 miles or just a mile. It is my freedom, my time to think, to de-stress and to explore. I may not be doing ultramarathons any more, but I am still a runner, and that makes me very happy.

EPILOGUE

When I returned from America in 2017, I was in such a bad place. I was down, but it turns out, not out. The doors to ultrarunning had all slammed shut for me, but that didn't mean I wouldn't find new ones to open. If you ever find yourself in a similar situation, having to give up the sport you love, don't despair. There will always be something else out there for you, even if you don't find it straight away. Keep looking and you never know what the future holds. I never expected to become a triathlete in my fifties or to find such joy and feelings of accomplishment from cycling and swimming. My swimming/tri coach Kevin believes I could even qualify to compete for GB in my age group in an international triathlon event if I keep putting the work in and keep improving. There is a long way to go to get to that stage, but it would be fantastic to represent my country in triathlon. I am currently enjoying training and racing when I feel like it without any pressure to be competitive. Never say never though!

The next challenge for me will be to complete a triathlon with an open-water swim. The thought of it terrifies me so

I have put off entering one, and it was taken out of my hands in 2020 with the Coronavirus pandemic resulting in cancelled races. But I know one day I will face my fears and give it a good try (or should that be tri?!). As children's author Dr Seuss aptly puts it: "You'll never be bored when you try something new. There's really no limit to what you can do."

MIMI'S SPORTING ACHIEVEMENTS SO FAR

2001

Thames Meander, 54-mile (87-km) race from Reading to London.

Marathon des Sables, 155-mile (249-km) six-day staged race in the Sahara Desert.

2002

Trailwalker UK, 62-mile (100-km) race over the South Downs from Queen Elizabeth Country Park, Hampshire, to Brighton racecourse, finished fastest mixed team.

2003

Marathon of Britain, 175-mile (282-km) seven-day staged race from Warwickshire to Nottingham, 3rd fastest female.

2004

Himalayan 100, 100-mile (161-km) five-day staged race, 3rd fastest female.

Rome Marathon, 26.2 miles (42.16 km). *PB: 3 hours 34 minutes*.

Grand Union Canal Race, 145 miles (233 km) non-stop from Birmingham to London, 2nd fastest female / 15th overall out of 23 finishers (54 runners started the race), finishing time 39 hours 39 minutes.

2005

Badwater Ultramarathon, 135 miles (217 km) starting in Death Valley and finishing in the Mount Witney Portals, USA, 6th fastest female, 1st Brit, 23rd overall, finishing time 41 hours, 5 minutes, 35 seconds.

Paris to London, 330 miles (531 km), including marathons in both cities.

2006

Kalahari Augrabies Extreme Marathon, 155-mile (249-km) self-sufficiency desert race over seven days, 1st female, 6th overall, finishing time 31 hours, 46 minutes.

Pennine Challenge 100, 62 miles (100 km), 1st female, 1st female veteran (age 40 and over), 4th overall out of eight finishers (29 competitors started the event), finishing time 30 hours, 34 minutes.

Libyan Challenge Master Trek, 120-mile (193-km) non-stop self-sufficiency desert race over four days, 1st female, 3rd overall.

Tring 2 Town, 45 miles (73 km) from London's Little Venice to Tring, 2nd female, 1st female veteran, finishing time 7 hours, 47 minutes.

2007

CHAMPION AND COURSE RECORD: *6633 Arctic Ultra*, a 352-mile (566-km) self-sufficiency race in the Arctic over eight days. I won in 143 hours, 23 minutes – just under six days, coming in 24 hours ahead of the next person and setting a course record.

Seni Extreme, 200-mile (322-km) non-stop race from Dudley, just north of Birmingham, to the ExCel Arena in London. I won in 67 hours, 13 minutes.

2008

FEMALE GUINNESS WORLD RECORD JOGLE: beginning in John o'Groats all the way to Land's End, 840 miles (1,352 km) in total in 12 days, 15 hours and 46 minutes.

Cape Odyssey, five-day staged race held in the Western Cape of South Africa run in teams of pairs. My team finished 53rd out of 164.

Atacama Crossing, 150-mile self-sufficiency staged race in the Atacama Desert, Chile, 1st female, 20th overall, finishing time 43 hours, 15 minutes.

Tring 2 Town 'Double', 80 miles (129 km), 2nd female, 1st female veteran.

Thames Path Challenge, 50-mile (80-km) race from Reading to Shepperton, with navigation as the Thames was flooded so we had to find our own routes, 2nd female in 7 hours, 48 minutes.

2009

FIRST FEMALE TO COMPLETE DOUBLE COMRADES: 56 miles (90 km) from Durban to Pietermaritzburg in 9 hours, 50 minutes, followed by joining in the official race to run back again in 10 hours, 40 minutes, covering a total of 112 miles (180 km).

The Druid's Challenge, 82-mile (132-km) three-day event along the Ridgeway, from Wiltshire to Buckinghamshire, 25th overall.

Kalahari Augrabies Extreme Marathon, 10th overall, 1st female, finishing time 27 hours, 5 minutes (4 minutes faster than in 2006).

Al Andalus Ultra Trail, 62-mile (100-km) five-day staged race in Spain, 8th overall, 1st female.

Tring 2 Town Double, 80 miles (129 km), 8th overall, 1st female, finishing time 12 hours, 42 minutes.

2010

FEMALE TREADMILL GUINNESS WORLD RECORD: furthest distance covered on a treadmill in seven days by a female, a total of 403.81 miles (649.87 km). This record has since been broken a number of times.

FEMALE COURSE RECORD GRAND UNION CANAL RACE: 145 miles (233 km) non-stop from Birmingham to London, 3rd overall, 1st female, setting a new course record for women in 28 hours and 12 minutes.

Namibian Desert Challenge, 136-mile (219-km) five-day self-sufficiency staged race, won overall in 25 hours and 23 minutes.

2011

FIRST FEMALE TO COMPLETE DOUBLE BADWATER: I ran the Badwater Ultramarathon (135 miles / 217 km), then climbed to the top of Mount Whitney (14,505 ft / 4,421 m above sea level, 11 miles / 17.7 km), then back down the mountain and all the way back to the start of the original race, a total distance of 292 miles (470 km). I finished in 108 hours and 10 minutes becoming the first British female to complete the double.

Spartathlon, 153-mile (246-km) non-stop race from Athens to Sparta in under 36 hours with cut-offs at every checkpoint. I finished 37th out of 285 starters (145 finishers), 1st Brit and 3rd female in a time of 32 hours, 33 minutes.

Glenmore 24 Trail Race, as many laps of the 4-mile (6.44-km) course as you can in 24 hours. I ran 112 miles, was 3rd overall and 1st female.

Ronda 101, 63-mile (101-km) trail race in Spain to be completed in 24 hours, 3rd female and 2nd female veteran, in 11 hours and 31 minutes.

Glasgow to Edinburgh Ultramarathon, 56 miles (90 km) along the canals, finished 11th overall and 1st female, finishing time 9 hours, 7 minutes.

2012

GUINNESS WORLD RECORD, THE FASTEST CROSSING ON FOOT OF IRELAND: started in Malin Head and finished at Mizen Head, a total of 345 miles (555 km) in three days, 15 hours, 36 minutes and 55 seconds.

Jungle Ultramarathon, 146-mile (235-km) six-day staged race in the jungle of Peru, 4th overall and 1st female, finishing time 32 hours, 49 minutes.

Viking Way Ultra, 148-mile (238-km) non-stop race starting at the Humber Bridge, Yorkshire, and finishing in Oakham, Rutland, 3rd overall and the first ever female to complete the course in 33 hours, 52 minutes.

Thames Path 100, 100-mile (161-km) non-stop race starting in Richmond, London, finishing in Oxford along the Thames Path, 7th overall, 1st female in a time of 18 hours, 50 minutes.

2013

FIRST PERSON TO COMPLETE DOUBLE GRAND UNION CANAL RACE: a total of 290 miles (467 km) from London to Birmingham and back again. I did the first leg in 31 hours and 50 minutes and the return journey (as part of the official race) in 36 hours, 49 minutes.

Mountain Ultra, 146-mile (235-km) five-day staged race in Colorado, USA, 2nd female, finishing time 33 hours, 15 minutes.

2014

1243 miles (1,968 km) on the Freedom Trail, run over 32 days in South Africa from Pietermaritzburg to Paarl, just outside Cape Town.

Cyprus Ultra, 135 miles (217 km) non-stop. I was the only finisher, setting a new course record of 41 hours, 34 minutes.

2015

Thames Path 100, (see 2012) 2nd female, finishing time 18 hours, 50 minutes.

Grand Union Canal Race, (see 2010) 1st female, finishing time 28 hours, 12 minutes.

Run the Rann, I took part in the inaugural 100-mile (161-km) non-stop event in a remote area of India, across salt flats, cliffs and through tonnes of thorny bushes, 2nd female, finishing time 39 hours, 55 minutes.

FIRST FEMALE TO COMPLETE THE DOUBLE SPARTATHLON: I took part in the 153-mile (246-km) non-stop race from Athens to Sparta with cut-offs at every checkpoint, finishing in 35 hours and 7 minutes. After a few hours' rest, I turned back to complete the course in reverse, running a total of 306 miles (492 km).

2016

Ice Ultramarathon, 143-mile (230-km) self-sufficiency race through Arctic Sweden, 4th overall, 1st female.

2017

GUINNESS WORLD RECORD ATTEMPT – COAST TO COAST ACROSS THE USA: starting in L.A., I set out to run 2,850 miles (4,587 km) to finish in New York, 53 days later. I reached 2,215.24 miles (3,565 km) in 40 days before I had to pull out with injury.

2018

Coast to Coast, 140-mile (225-km) ride from Whitehaven, Cumbria, to Tynmouth, Tyne and Wear, completed in 2.5 days.

Deloitte Ride Across Britain, a 980-mile (1,577-km) ride held over nine days from Land's End to John o'Groats.

2019

Hell of the Ashdown, a 66.5-mile (107-km) cycle sportive over a testing route through Kent and Sussex, completed in 5 hours and 35 minutes.

Audax Event, a 192-mile (309-km) ride from Chalfont St Peter, Buckinghamshire, to Fordingbridge, Hampshire and back.

Castle 100, a charity bike ride through the Kent countryside taking in the North Downs.

Cranbrook Sprint Triathlon, 300 m (328 yd) pool swim, 21 km (13 mile) cycle and 5 km (3.1 mile) run, first female V55, finishing time 1 hour, 30 minutes and 51 seconds.

Prudential Ride London, a 100-mile (161-km) route on closed roads starting at the Queen Elizabeth Olympic Park, Stratford, out to Surrey passing over Box Hill before finishing on The Mall in central London.

Cycling the Pacific Coast Highway, 1,850 miles (2,977 km) from Vancouver, Canada, to the Mexican border in California, USA, carrying all my kit on the bike, camping along the way, completed in 25 days.

2020

No races due to events being cancelled because of the Coronavirus pandemic.

2021

Watch this space! Follow me on Twitter and Instagram @marvellousmimi and like my Facebook page, Mimi Anderson – endurance athlete, for training and race updates. I also blog regularly at my website, www.marvellousmimi.com.

ACKNOWLEDGEMENTS

This book is largely about my US world record attempt, which was only made possible thanks to my amazing crew. Thank you from the top to the bottom of my heart for giving up your time to come and support me. You really are without doubt the best team of people in the entire world and I love each and every one of you for what you have done for me. Although we didn't get the outcome we all wanted, it really was an adventure and a half. Each of you brought your own special talents to the team, which is why it worked so well, enabling me to do my job of running without having to think about anything else.

Jenny, you led the team brilliantly, it must have been extremely tough but you organized doctors, hospitals, trainers and a huge amount more without fuss: everything just got done.

Jan, what can I say about your food – simply delicious! As someone who doesn't particularly enjoy eating even I found myself looking forward to my dinner in the evenings!

ACKNOWLEDGEMENTS

Becky and Paul, you guys knew me best of all and it was an honour to have you there for the first three weeks of the run, giving up your honeymoon and coming on a runningmoon!

Sophie, you are a remarkable young lady who has a massive heart (and a big brain!). You will go a long way in your life, of that I have no doubt. If anyone would like to read about Sophie's incredible run across Scandinavia, then I recommend her book, *Rundinavia*.

Darren, you arrived to be part of a mad group of people who were already sleep-deprived and slotted in brilliantly. And as for your spaghetti – yummy!

Fiona, Beccy and Nicola, you ladies were without a doubt an essential part of my everyday life, thank you, each of you were brilliant.

Tim, thank you for being there and staying on. I don't think even now you have any idea how much that means to me.

To Carol and Susie from Scrumptious Productions, thank you for taking such an interest in my story and for joining us on the journey across America. It wouldn't have been the same without you both; you became integral members of the team and helped me keep going on numerous occasions. I can't wait to watch the finished documentary. I know it will have me in floods of tears but also bring back a lot of happy memories. If you would like to watch it, please keep an eye on my social media pages (as listed below) for updates on how and when it will be broadcast.

I'm also very grateful to James Manclark for his financial support, and to my sponsors: VW America, Qubit, Noxgear, X-Bionic, Hoka OneOne, The Ultrarunning Marathon Store, Rocktape, Likeys, ++Suunto, Truestart Coffee and Chase-Life for everything they provided to help me. Thank you.

To my coach Ray Zahab, thank you for your support and advice and for getting me in the best possible shape to attempt to run nearly 3,000 miles.

Thank you to everyone who supported me along the way and donated to my charities Marie Curie and Free to Run. Thanks to you, I raised a total of £7,706.84. My JustGiving page is no longer active, but you can still support and find out more about these charities via their websites: mariecurie.org.uk and freetorun.org

When it comes to my new adventures in cycling, swimming and triathlon, thank you to my friends at Weald Tri Club for your support, friendship and encouragement. I can't recommend joining such clubs enough, never think you are not good enough to become a member as they cater for everyone.

To my swimming and triathlon coach Kevin Draper, thank you so much for your incredible patience and excellent teaching. I can't believe how far I have come, and I wouldn't have been able to do it without you.

And, of course, a huge thank you to my wonderful family and friends (too many of you to name here) for always being there for me.

ACKNOWLEDGEMENTS

My ghostwriter, Lucy Waterlow, and I would like to thank all the team at Summersdale for believing in my story and allowing me to tell it in not one but two books! I have been overwhelmed by the response to my first book *Beyond Impossible*. I love hearing how it has inspired people to take up running, and how it has helped people dealing with eating disorders. I hope this book will do the same by perhaps encouraging more people to try cycling, swimming and triathlon too. You never know what you are capable of until you try.

And finally thank you, the reader, I really hope you have enjoyed sharing my journey via my books. I would love to know what you think. Get in touch via Twitter and Instagram @marvellousmimi or my Facebook page, Mimi Anderson – endurance athlete. You could also leave a review on the Limitless Amazon page.

Have you enjoyed this book?

If so, why not write a review on your favourite website?

If you're interested in finding out more about our books,
find us on Facebook at **Summersdale Publishers** and follow
us on Twitter at **@Summersdale**.

Thanks very much for buying this Summersdale book.

www.summersdale.com